Translational Application of Artificial Intelligence in Healthcare

In the era of 'Algorithmic Medicine', the integration of Artificial Intelligence (AI) in healthcare holds immense potential to address critical challenges faced by the industry.

Drawing upon the expertise and experience of the authors in medicine, data science, medical informatics, administration, and entrepreneurship, this textbook goes beyond theoretical discussions to outline practical steps for transitioning AI from the experimental phase to real-time clinical integration. Using the Translational Science methodology, each chapter of the book concisely and clearly addresses the key issues associated with AI implementation in healthcare. Covering technical, clinical, ethical, regulatory, and legal considerations, the authors present evidence-based solutions and frameworks to overcome these challenges.

Engaging case studies and a literature review of peer-reviewed studies and official documents from reputed organizations provide a balanced perspective, bridging the gap between AI research and actual clinical practice.

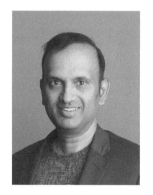

Sandeep Reddy is an Artificial Intelligence (AI) in healthcare researcher based at the Deakin School of Medicine, as well as being the founder/chairman of Centre for Advancement of Translational AI in Medicine, a healthcare-focused AI entity. He is also a certified health informatician and World Health Organization–recognised digital health expert. He has a medical and healthcare management background and has completed machine learning/health informatics training from various sources. He is currently engaged in research about the safety, quality and explainability of the application of AI in healthcare delivery, in addition to developing AI models to treat and manage chronic diseases. He has also authored several articles and books about the use of AI in medicine. Further, he has set up local and international forums to promote the use of AI in healthcare and sits on various international committees which focus on this issue.

ANALYTICS AND AI FOR HEALTHCARE

Artificial Intelligence (AI) and analytics are increasingly being applied to various healthcare settings. AI and analytics are salient to facilitate better understanding and identifying key insights from healthcare data in many areas of practice and enquiry including at the genomic, individual, hospital, community and/or population levels. The Chapman & Hall/CRC Press Analytics and AI in Healthcare Series aims to help professionals upskill and leverage the techniques, tools, technologies and tactics of analytics and AI to achieve better healthcare delivery, access, and outcomes. The series covers all areas of analytics and AI as applied to healthcare. It will look at critical areas including prevention, prediction, diagnosis, treatment, monitoring, rehabilitation and survivorship.

ABOUT THE SERIES EDITOR

Professor Nilmini Wickramasinghe *is Professor of Digital Health and the Deputy Director of the Iverson Health Innovation Research Institute at Swinburne University of Technology, Australia and is inaugural Professor – Director Health Informatics Management at Epworth HealthCare, Victoria, Australia. She also holds honorary research professor positions at the Peter MacCallum Cancer Centre, Murdoch Children's Research Institute and Northern Health. For over 20 years, Professor Wickramasinghe has been researching and teaching within the health informatics/digital health domain. She was awarded the prestigious Alexander von Humboldt award in recognition of her outstanding contribution to digital health.*

Explainable AI in Healthcare
Mehul S. Raval, Mohendra Roy, Tolga Kaya & Rupal A. Kapdi

Data Analysis in Medicine and Health Using R
Kamarul Imran Musa, Wan Nor Arifin Wan Mansor & Tengku Muhammad Hanis

Data Driven Science for Clinically Actionable Knowledge in Diseases
Quang Vinh Nguyen, Paul J. Kennedy, Simeon J. Simoff & Daniel R. Catchpoole

Translational Application of Artificial Intelligence in Healthcare
-A Textbook
Edited by Sandeep Reddy

For more information about this series please visit: https://www.routledge.com/analytics-and-ai-for-healthcare/book-series/Aforhealth

This book provides a very readable introduction into our current understanding of all these issues and affords the opportunity for non-AI experts to appreciate how AI can improve clinical care while being made aware of its current limitations and how these may be overcome.

Professor Ian Scott, *Director of Internal Medicine and Clinical Epidemiology, Princess Alexandra Hospital; Professor of Medicine, University of Queensland*

This book is essential because it begins to delineate that pathway to implementation, guiding readers to consider issues beyond predictive performance as they develop the AI applications of the future.

Professor Wendy W. Chapman, *Director of the Centre for Digital Transformation of Health, University of Melbourne*

Advances in technology have always been a driver for improved delivery of healthcare. The application of AI in healthcare has the potential to be the driver that will lead to a more effective and efficient healthcare delivery system. This book provides a very lucid overview of the potential applications and benefits, and also addresses the potential challenges in the adoption of AI in healthcare. A sound grounding and understanding of the potential applications of AI will empower clinicians and scientists to adapt and hopefully expand the scope of its application.

Girish Nair, *Director of Functional Neurosurgery, The Royal Melbourne Hospital and Head of Unit of Neurosurgery, Western Health*

The hardest part of innovation is not invention but the implementation of new technology. Moreover, clinical medicine, where one mistake may affect the mortality of innumerable people, is one of the most difficult fields to implement emerging technologies. Although it won't teach us the best racing line for the podium, this book shows us the starting grid of the circuit for the ones who want to achieve innovation.

Tomohiro Kuroda, *CIO of Kyoto University Hospital, Director of the Center for Digital Transformation of Healthcare, Professor of Graduate School of Medicine, Professor of Graduate School of Informatics, Kyoto University*

Translational Application of Artificial Intelligence in Healthcare

-A Textbook

Edited by
Sandeep Reddy

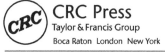

CRC Press
Taylor & Francis Group
Boca Raton London New York

CRC Press is an imprint of the
Taylor & Francis Group, an **informa** business
A CHAPMAN & HALL BOOK

Cover design credit: © Shutterstock

First edition published 2024
by CRC Press
2385 NW Executive Center Drive, Suite 320, Boca Raton FL 33431

and by CRC Press
4 Park Square, Milton Park, Abingdon, Oxon, OX14 4RN

CRC Press is an imprint of Taylor & Francis Group, LLC

© 2024 selection and editorial matter, Sandeep Reddy; individual chapters, the contributors

ISBN: 978-1-032-20090-3 (hbk)
ISBN: 978-1-032-20088-0 (pbk)
ISBN: 978-1-003-26215-2 (ebk)

DOI: 10.1201/9781003262152

Typeset in Palatino
by SPi Technologies India Pvt Ltd (Straive)

Contents

Contributors

Dr Bart Geerts
Healthplus.AI
Amsterdam, Netherlands

Dr Sandra Johnson
University of Sydney School of Medicine
Sydney, Australia

Dr Vince Madai
Charité Universitätsmedizin
Berlin, Germany

Dr Dwarikanath Mahapatra
Inception AI
Abu Dhabi, UAE

Dr Piyush Mathur
Cleveland Clinic
Cleveland, OH, USA

Dr Francis Papay
Cleveland Clinic
Cleveland, OH, USA

Dr Sandeep Reddy
Deakin School of Medicine
Geelong, Australia

Dr Sonika Tyagi
RMIT
Melbourne, Australia

Dr Stephen Whebell
Townsville Hospital
Townsville, Australia

Dr Joe Zhang
Imperial College London
London, UK

Abbreviations

AI   Artificial Intelligence

A branch of computer science that deals with the creation of intelligent agents, which are systems that can reason, learn, and act autonomously.

CDS   Clinical Decision Support

A type of deep learning algorithm that is used for natural language processing and speech recognition.

CNN   Convolutional Neural Network

A type of deep learning algorithm that is used for image recognition and natural language processing.

DL   Deep Learning

A type of machine learning that uses artificial neural networks to learn from data.

ML   Machine Learning

A subset of AI that allows computers to learn without being explicitly programmed.

PH   Personalized Health

A type of AI that is used to tailor healthcare interventions to individual patients.

RD   Drug Discovery

A type of AI that is used to identify new drug targets and design new drugs.

1

An Introduction to Artificial Intelligence

Sandeep Reddy

Deakin School of Medicine, Geelong, Australia

LEARNING OBJECTIVES

- Describe what AI is
- Discuss the various categories of AI
- Describe the various models of AI
- Explain how AI is used in healthcare
- Identify the challenges in the adoption of AI in healthcare

Introduction

We currently live in the age of Big Data (Reddy & Cooper, 2021). Over the past few decades, this has been characterized by exponential production, storage, and data sharing. Big data has been described as "high-volume, high-velocity and/or high-variety" information that requires novel and efficient analysis to gain valuable insights (Cappa et al., 2021). The latter part of the description is particularly relevant to the discussion here. As data production has increased significantly, the manual processing of such data to yield actionable insights has become impractical (Reddy & Cooper, 2021). Automated analysis of such data through computational reasoning frameworks has become a more attractive and practical proposition. Artificial Intelligence (AI), a computational reasoning framework, has emerged as a leading technology in the field of data science. AI is an umbrella term representing a group of techniques that replicate aspects of human intelligence, including visual perception, speech recognition and judgement (Lidströmer et al., 2021). While AI is one of the newest fields of engineering, the introduction of the concept can be traced back hundreds of years (Reddy, 2018). However, AI as a formal discipline emerged only in the 1950s. Since then, AI has been used across various sectors and disciplines, including, pertinent to this book, in healthcare, to automate or semi-automate the processing of data and resultant tasks (Reddy & Cooper, 2021).

In healthcare, obtaining information early in the disease process and intervening early and effectively is critical to good medical practice and the achievement of good patient outcomes. Having access to an automated system, trained on relevant data, recognising meaningful relationships intrinsic to the data, and supporting clinical decision-making would significantly enhance the practice of medicine (Ganguli et al., n.d.; GAO, 2020). The current generation of AI algorithms is far more advanced in their capacity to self-learn and mirror human knowledge than the previous generations (Jordan & Mithcell, 2015). Many AI applications are now trained by using examples of input–output behaviour rather than the manual programming of all anticipated responses. This process has enabled AI's broader and yet deeper application in intense data environments such as medicine. With such potential for widespread use comes the opportunity and the technical, medical, ethical, legal, and social challenges (Desai, 2020). Over this chapter and those which follow, we will introduce the reader to fundamental concepts of AI, its application in healthcare, the opportunities, the issues associated with AI's implementation in healthcare and various solutions to address these issues.

Description of AI

Considering the popularity and complexity of AI, it is no wonder that one comes across myriad descriptions. However, most of these descriptions have some common themes, including machines or computers, synthetic intelligence, and intelligent agents (Jordan & Mithcell, 2015; Lidströmer et al., 2021; Reddy, 2018). A great starting point in describing or defining AI is understanding its fundamental objective, i.e., for machines to replicate or simulate human-level intelligence (Reddy, 2018). While the objective seems simple, the process is incredibly complex and not standardized, leading to difficulties in describing AI. However, the 'intelligent agent' is critical in achieving 'artificial' intelligence. These agents can demonstrate intelligent behaviour, which means they are not only capable of perception of their environment but also can undertake practical reasoning and suitable action to achieve their goals. Thus, a definition of AI could be *'the science of making intelligent machines'*. This definition corresponds to how it had been envisaged by John McCarthy, one of the founding fathers of modern AI (Reddy et al., 2019). Another approach to defining AI is to consider the actions of AI, such as emulating features of human intelligence (including reasoning, complex task processing, decision-making, communication, knowledge representation and so forth) and the process requiring utilization of computer programming and machines. Based on this, one could also define AI as 'machines simulating human intelligence'.

AI Categories

As with the definition of AI, one can come across various categories of AI. Some categories relate to functionalities; others are based on capabilities and applications (Bartneck et al., 2021a; Lidströmer et al., 2021; Reddy, 2018). However, others classify AI based on its application areas, such as natural language processing, computer vision, robotics and so on (Jordan & Mithcell, 2015; Reddy et al., 2019). For the purpose of this introductory chapter, we consider all these classifications. In the first categorization, we describe AI

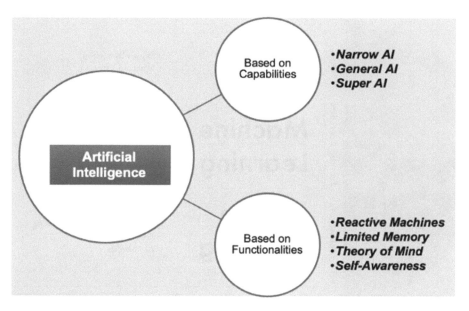

FIGURE 1.1
Artificial intelligence (AI) categories based on capabilities and functionalities.

(Source: Author.)

based on its capabilities and functions (Figure 1.1). From a capability point of view, when AI can only perform a specific task or, in other words, a very defined activity, it is termed 'Narrow AI'. Some also refer to this as 'Weak AI' (Bartneck et al., 2021b). When AI can undertake any intellectual task at the level of humans, then it is termed 'General AI'. This term indicates that AI can generalize and represent learning across several cognitive functions. This category is also called 'Strong AI' (Bartneck et al., 2021b; Butz, 2021). On the other hand, 'Super AI' is when machines can exceed the level of human intelligence and perform tasks better than humans. Currently, both general and super AI are theoretical concepts, and some scientists doubt these two forms of AI are feasible (Fjelland, 2020). Nevertheless, others speculate that humans may not have control over super AI due to fundamental limits intrinsic to computing.

We have four categories when we consider AI based on its functionalities commencing with the basic functioning of AI to the most advanced level where AI has conscious-ness (Hintze, 2016). The first category, as per this stratification, is 'Reactive Machines', where you have fundamental AI systems that are purely reactive and incapable of form-ing memories or making decisions based on past experiences. Here the computer per-ceives and acts concerning what it sees but does not rely on the internal representation of the world. The next category is a step up and is called 'Limited Memory'. Here the machine can store past experiences and limited data for a short period. The machine can investigate the past, but only for a transitory period. 'Theory of Mind', the next group-ing, separates the status of AI from what many are aiming for AI to be (Cuzzolin et al., 2020). Here, machines can understand human emotions and interact with them socially. The machines can form representations of the world and its entities and lead to social interactions. This representation is a critical step for machines to progress to the level

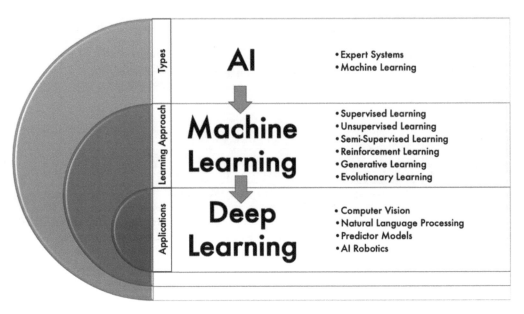

FIGURE 1.2
AI categories based on learning approaches and applications.

(Source: Author.)

of humans. The final classification, and a significant step for AI, is to develop its awareness, consciousness, and sentiments. This category is termed 'Self-Awareness'. Having self-awareness means machines can form representations of themselves and potentially build other machines with self-awareness. Currently, both 'Theory of Mind' and 'Self-Awareness' are theoretical concepts without any evidence of the development of such machines (Hintze, 2016).

Another way to group AI is based on the type of algorithms or models used. Based on this, AI can be classified into the two currently used models: 'Expert Systems' and 'Machine Learning' (Figure 1.2).

Expert Systems

For decades, the predominant approach in AI was the use of expert systems or knowledge-based systems (Lidströmer et al., 2021; Reddy, 2018). This approach replaced the previous emphasis on identifying universal methods for problem-solving with focusing on representation and solving specific problems using the knowledge of experts (Jordan & Mithcell, 2015; Tan, 2017). Thus, expert systems were meant to embody the knowledge of a human expert and assist non-experts in investigating a relevant problem or field (Tan, 2017). The three main components of an expert system include

    a) a knowledge base of facts associated with the domain, and heuristics (problem-solving approach)

b) an inference process for utilising the knowledge base to identify a solution for the problem, and

c) a global database to keep track of the problem status, the input data for the specific problem and a history of associated activity. In other words, this component is the working memory of the system.

When introduced in the 1960s, expert systems became one of the truly successful forms of AI (Tan, 2017). Expert systems then went on to proliferate and predominate in the 1980s. They could be installed and run on any computer hardware, provide a higher level of expertise than a human expert, and explain how the problem was solved and was fast in most instances. However, they also presented several challenges, the most typical being knowledge acquisition. Obtaining the knowledge and time of human experts to develop and design the systems proved very challenging. So were the other problems associated with the life cycle of expert systems like integration, access to large databases and performance. These problems were such that, even though improved expert systems continue to be used nowadays, when machine learning, which relied less on knowledge engineering, emerged (Jordan & Mithcell, 2015), expert systems were gradually replaced with machine learning methods.

Machine Learning

The introduction of machine learning approaches allowed AI programmers to train a system through examples of desired input–output behaviour rather than program the system manually by anticipating the desired response to all possible inputs as with expert systems (Bi et al., 2019). In other words, machine learning would allow learning of behaviour not explicitly programmed into the system, The behaviour is learnt based on the data provided, by minimising the error between the current action and the desired one, and a feedback approach that facilitates the machine to self-recognise issues and improve performance.

Machine learning as a discipline is focused on two critical computational questions: a) How can one develop computer systems that automatically improve through experience? and b) What laws govern all learning systems including humans, organizations, and computers? (Jordan & Mithcell, 2015) Machine learning has rapidly developed, particularly over the past two decades from being a novel area to an established technology with myriad applications including for commercial use. Within AI, machine learning has become the predominant approach and is used to develop software for computer vision, speech recognition, natural language processing, robotics, and data mining. As outlined in Figure 1.2, machine learning has several subcategories, some of which are profiled below.

Supervised Learning

Machine learning can be broadly classified based on whether the approach to learning is supervised or unsupervised. In supervised learning, the machine learning models form their predictions via learned mapping (Bartneck et al., 2021b). This means that the value of the outcome or dependent variable is known for each observation (Lidströmer et al., 2021). The data with specified outcomes is termed labelled data. Many popular machine learning algorithms, including linear and logistic regression, decision trees, support vector machines and neural networks, adopt this approach. In deep neural networks, the internal layers can be considered providing the learned representations of the input data and much of practical successes of deep learning has been due to supervised learning discovering such representations (Bengio et al., 2021; LeCun et al., 2015).

Unsupervised Learning

In unsupervised learning, the model aims to identify natural relationships and groupings within the available data without referring to any outcome (Bi et al., 2019). This means the models discover useful representation of the input without the need for labelled data. The unsupervised approach attempts to identify unspecified subgroups that share similar characteristics within the data. Commonly used unsupervised learning algorithms are clustering algorithms, which group observations based on the similarity of data characteristics. Examples of such algorithms include k-means clustering and clustering using Gaussian mixture models.

In another type of machine learning called 'Semi-supervised Learning', the training involves both labelled and unlabelled data (Bi et al., 2019). When labelling data becomes time-consuming and expensive, a limited amount of labelled data is combined with a large amount of unlabelled data to derive optimal model performance. This type of machine learning has similarities to statistical techniques that focus on imputing missing outcomes.

Reinforcement Learning

This is a newer form of machine learning, in which reward functions are maximized based on the actions undertaken by the agent (Bi et al., 2019; Heidrich-Meisner et al., 2007). To train the agent, a trial-and-error approach is adopted to eventually arrive at optimal decision-making. Instead of training with examples outlining correct output for a given input, the training data provides an indication of whether the action undertaken was correct or not. Reinforcement learning algorithms typically make us of control-theory, including elements such as policy iteration, value iteration, roll outs and variance reduction (Heidrich-Meisner et al., 2007).

Deep Learning

Deep learning is an advanced form of machine learning that has an ability to automate feature extraction and analyse high dimensional data, thus advancing the field of AI like no other algorithm (Bengio et al., 2021). Computational neural networks, which form the basis of deep learning, are inspired by the architecture and signalling behaviour of biological neural networks (Bi et al., 2019; Lidströmer et al., 2021). The 'artificial' neural networks comprise of a population of neurons interconnected with each other through complex signalling pathways (Figure 1.3). The structure consists of a layer of neurons

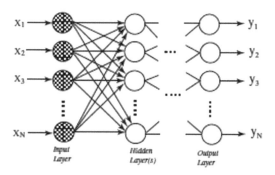

FIGURE 1.3
Neural network basic architecture.

(Source: Lidströmer et al., 2021.)

connected with each other by edges and grouped into an input layer, one or more mid-dle 'hidden' layers and an output later. The structure is used to analyse complex inter-actions between a group of measurable covariates to predict an outcome (Lidströmer et al., 2021).

There are many classes of deep learning algorithms but a notable class that has revo-lutionized and dominated computer vision is the convolutional neural network (CNN) (Lidströmer et al., 2021; Yamashita et al., 2018). This algorithmic class has been designed to learn spatial hierarchies automatically and adaptively via back propagation. They rely on a mathematical operation called convolution instead of general matrix multiplication. The class has been specifically designed to analyse pixel data, so very suited for image recognition and processing. The algorithmic structure typically comprises of three types of layers: convolution, pooling, and fully connected layer. With each layer, the network increases in its complexity (Figure 1.4) by identifying greater portions of the relevant image. As the image data progresses through the layers, the algorithm identifies larger elements of the image until it finally identifies the target area (Yamashita et al., 2018).

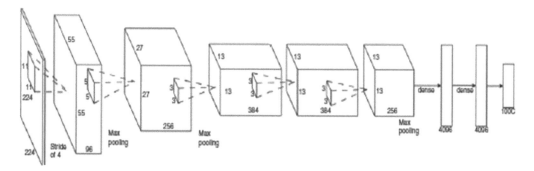

FIGURE 1.4
Convolutional neural network architecture with a fully connected dense layer.

(Source: Lidströmer et al., 2021.)

Transformers

One recent development with neural networks concerns transformers. These algorithms are based on a self-attention mechanism, which works particularly well for language understanding (Vaswani et al., 2017). Like other neural networks, transformers are designed to process sequential input data; however, unlike other neural networks, transformers process all the input simultaneously. The attention mechanism enables every element in the input data to connect to every other element (Figure 1.5). This aspect allows parallelization and the reduction of training times. Transformers have now become the basis for large language models or foundational models, which are

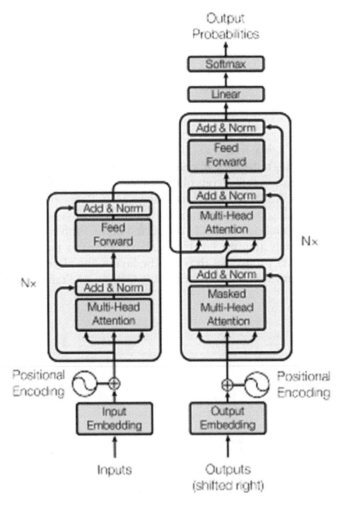

FIGURE 1.5
Transformer model architecture.

(Source: Vaswani et al., 2017.)

trained on hundreds of billions of words and can analyse and predict text to an unsettling degree (Luitse & Denkena, 2021).

Large Language Models

Large Language Models (LLMs) are neural network models, based on the afore discussed transformer architecture, that can carry on a dialog (Gruetzemacher & Paradice, 2022). These LLMs are self-supervised and can perform many different language tasks, exhibiting new language skills with just a few examples (Agrawal et al., 2022). They can generate natural language texts based on a given input such as a prompt, a question, or a document. Using word representations to encode the semantics of words in a language, statistical language models can be created to model the probability of word occurrence in sentences (see Figure 1.6). LLMs are probability distributions of sequences of words that are useful for problems that require the prediction of the next word in a sequence given the previous words. LLMs have been trained on massive amounts of text data from various sources such as the internet, books, news articles, and social media posts. LLMs have shown remarkable capabilities in generating coherent, fluent, and diverse texts across different domains and tasks such as writing stories, summarizing articles, answering questions, and creating chatbots (Agrawal et al., 2022; Gilson et al., 2023; Liebrenz et al., 2023; Patel & Lam, 2023).

Applications of AI

AI techniques have now clearly moved from the academic environment to real-world applications (Litman, 2021). The permeation of AI across multiple sectors, including banking, retail, social media, television, and of course healthcare, has demonstrated its

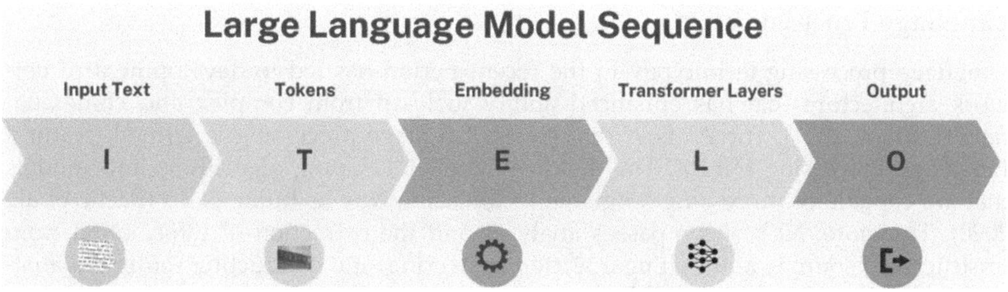

FIGURE 1.6
Large language model architecture.

(Source: Author.)

real-world utility (Zhang, 2021). AI is now used in these industries for audio-processing, facial or object recognition recommender systems, predictive analysis and, in certain instances, a combination of these processes. The performance of AI models in these instances is based on training in hundreds, thousands and even millions of data points that could be either structured or unstructured. The standard of AI, in certain conditions, is that its performance cannot be distinguished from humans. This indicates potential for AI to be scaled up or expanded to new avenues that are socially beneficial (Litman, 2021; Zhang, 2021).

Image Processing

AI-enabled image processing is now widespread with uses ranging from facial detection to generating photo-realistic images (Litman, 2021). The field of AI behind this is termed 'Computer Vision' (Zhang, 2021). This field introduced in the 1960s has now matured to a great extent. The common tasks of computer vision include object recognition, pose estimation and semantic segmentation amongst others. Some examples of the application of computer vision include medical image analysis, satellite imagery analysis, facial recognition systems, autonomous driving systems and defective part detection in manufacturing.

Since 2010s, computer vision has transitioned from use of classical machine learning techniques to deep learning (Montagnon et al., 2020). This development coupled with availability of powerful parallel computing hardware enabled through graphical processing units has industrialized image processing. Not only the training time for image processing has now reduced but also the performance of the relevant AI models has significantly improved (Zhang, 2021). However, now the performance of popular image processing models has flattened vis a vis available benchmarks necessitating new and harder benchmarks to assess their performance.

Language Processing

Language processing technology in the recent period has led to development of network architecture that has enhanced ability to learn from complex and contextual data (Litman, 2021). The AI field that covers language processing is termed 'Natural Language Processing (NLP)'. This field involves developing algorithms and models that are capable of processing language in the same way as humans do (Baclic et al., 2020). Therefore, NLP encompasses analyses and the extraction of information from unstructured sources, automating question answering, and conducting sentiment analysis and text summarization. NLP commenced in the 1950s as an intersecting discipline between AI and linguistics (Zhang, 2021). Current NLP borrows from several diverse fields and has allowed it to capture and model complex linguistic relationships and concepts. Modern NLP platforms are based on models refined through machine learning techniques, especially deep learning techniques. The models learn about how words are used in context by sifting through patterns that occur in natural text (Litman, 2021; Zhang, 2021). Some of the advanced NLP models consist of billions of tuneable parameters and are capable of processing unprecedented quantities of information. Further, several of these models can generate passages of texts that sometimes cannot be distinguished from human-generated text. However, it must be noted that these models are incapable of deep understanding of the texts they process. Current NLP applications include machine translation, text classification, speech recognition, writing aids and chatbots (Litman, 2021).

LLMs are now being considered for use in healthcare (Agrawal et al., 2022; Chen & Baxter, 2022; Patel & Lam, 2023; Yang et al., 2022). One of the most common applications of LLMs in healthcare is clinical note extraction (Agrawal et al., 2022; Patel & Lam, 2023). Clinical notes are written records of patient encounters that contain valuable information for diagnosis, treatment planning, and billing purposes. However, clinical notes are often unstructured, incomplete, inconsistent, and noisy, making it difficult for humans and machines to process and analyse them. LLMs can help extract important data from clinical notes such as symptoms, diagnoses, medications, procedures, and outcomes. This can assist with personalized medicine by providing tailored recommendations based on individual patient profiles. However, LLMs also pose significant challenges and risks when applied to sensitive and critical domains such as healthcare (Józefowicz et al., 2016; The Lancet Digital, 2023). Healthcare is a domain that requires high levels of accuracy, reliability, and ethics from any system that interacts with human health data and outcomes. Therefore, evaluating LLMs in the context of healthcare is crucial to ensure their quality, safety, and responsibility.

Robotics and AI

It is pertinent in this introductory chapter to discuss robotics and its relationship with AI. Robotics is an engineering branch that involves the design, development, and operation of robots (Ingrand & Ghallab, 2017). The discipline overlaps with many fields, including AI. In fact, recent years have witnessed an increasing convergence of AI and robotics. The reason for this was the optimization of the level of autonomy of robots through learning about its environment. The autonomy of a robot can be characterized by its level of perception, planning and execution (Figure 1.7) (Ingrand & Ghallab, 2017). This autonomy, coupled with intelligence (derived from AI) as measured by the robot's capacity to predict the future, plan a task, and interact with the environment, can push robots closer to human-level functioning. However, at this stage of development this level of functioning has proven difficult to achieve. At the time of writing, the most popular robot in medicine is a surgical robot which uses computer vision to capture images and an advanced motion control system to replicate the movements of a human arm (Reddy, 2018). In the future, more autonomous robots will allow for surgeries to be independently conducted by robots. Robots have also been used for transporting supplies and cleaning and disinfection in hospitals, for prosthetics and rehabilitation, and for social companionship.

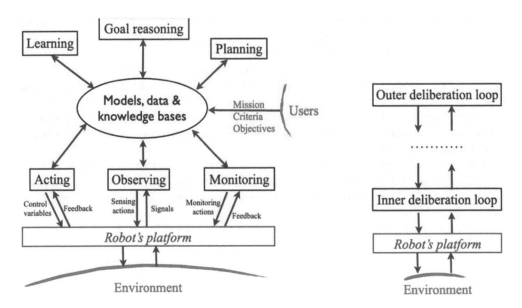

FIGURE 1.7
Deliberation functions in a robot.

(Source: Ingrand & Ghallab, 2017.)

Use of AI in Healthcare

Now that we have used this chapter to review the nature of AI and outline its separate categories, the rest of the book gives a detailed outline of AI's application in healthcare. To herald this description, here an overview of this application is presented. Contemporary approaches to AI separate it from the approaches of previous generations, which require mechanical or rule-based formulations (Jordan & Mithcell, 2015; Tan, 2017). The ability to autonomously generate rules has enabled the broader applicability of AI in healthcare. In addition, technical infrastructure such as AI chips and cloud computing to run advanced machine learning models like neural networks has supported the implementation of AI in healthcare (Reddy et al., 2019). AI is now widely considered to have the potential to have a profound impact on healthcare service planning and delivery (Lidströmer et al., 2021). In addition to improving treatment outcomes, AI is said to have the possibility to reduce the administrative burden for healthcare providers and increase the efficiency of delivering healthcare (Reddy et al., 2019). These outcomes can also result in the reduction of currently burgeoning costs in providing healthcare. Of the various available AI techniques, machine learning has had the greatest impact on furthering the use of AI in healthcare (Adlung et al., 2021; Jordan & Mithcell, 2015). Machine learning applications, including both clinical and administrative functions, have been used across the healthcare spectrum (Aung et al., 2021). Machine learning models have been used in the clinical environment to diagnose, prognosis, and treat patients (see Figure 1.8 and Case Study 1).

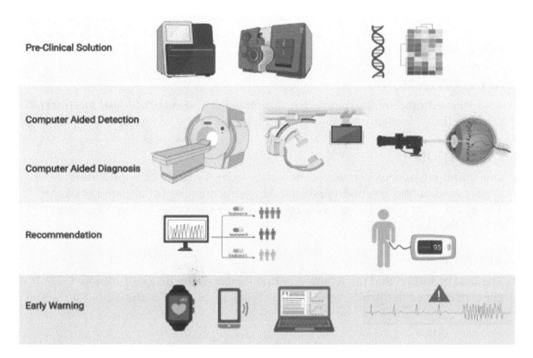

FIGURE 1.8
Machine learning applications in healthcare.

(Source: Adlung et al., 2021.)

A further detailed review of how AI and machine learning are used in healthcare is presented in the next chapter. Nevertheless, it is essential to mention here that we are still in the early days for the application of AI in healthcare. There is not yet the widespread adoption of AI to deliver healthcare, whether in clinical or administrative areas. Also, as the later chapters describe, a number of clinical, ethical, legal, and social concerns are potentially associated with the use of AI in all areas (Reddy et al., 2020; Reddy et al., 2021). However, concerted efforts are currently being made by researchers, clinicians, and policy makers to address these concerns and support the adoption of AI in healthcare (Bajwa et al., 2021; GAO, 2020).

CASE STUDY 1   A RANDOMIZED CLINICAL TRIAL OF AI ENABLED ELECTROCARDIOGRAMS FOR THE IDENTIFICATION OF LOW EJECTION FRACTION (YAO ET AL., 2021)

INTRODUCTION

Asymptomatic left ventricular systolic dysfunction confers a 6.5-fold increased risk of clinical heart failure (HF) and a 1.6-fold increased risk of all-cause mortality. While guideline-recommended therapies can reduce the risk of HF progression and mortality, low ejection fraction (EF) is often undiagnosed leading to missed treatment opportunities.

AI INTERVENTION

A supervised machine learning algorithm utilising a standard 12-lead electrocardiogram (ECG) to identify patients with a high likelihood of low EF.

EVALUATION

One hundred twenty primary care teams from 45 healthcare providers were cluster-randomized to enter either the AI intervention or usual patterns of care. The primary outcome being assessed was a new diagnosis of low EF within 90 days of the ECG.

RESULTS

The trial identified that the AI intervention increased the diagnosis of low EF (2.1 per cent increase in the intervention arm versus 1.6 per cent in the control arm).

The Future of AI

Recent developments in AI have propelled the adoption of computer-based reasoning in medicine (Reddy, 2018; Reddy & Cooper, 2021). Certain studies have demonstrated the accuracy of AI applications and illustrated how they meet the performance of human clinicians and, in some other instances, actually exceed the performance (Bajwa et al., 2021; GAO, 2020; Yao et al., 2021). Yet, there is a lack of widespread adoption of AI applications in clinical medicine, nor is there any active endorsement of their use by clinical bodies (Madai & Higgins, 2021). Further, concerns about the transparency and biases of AI applications persist (Reddy et al., 2020). However, considering some of the intractable problems faced by health services and healthcare, AI presents a novel and extraordinary opportunity to improve healthcare delivery and outcomes (Reddy, 2020a). Unlike previous and other technologies, the potential of AI to integrate into existing infrastructure and augment the performance of human clinicians is both clear and promising. To enable the better adoption of AI in medicine and realize its potential, it is necessary for there to be a combined effort on the part of researchers, clinicians, policy makers, and software developers to address the teething problems. In the end, the technical issues that relate to AI software development and integration in healthcare may not be as difficult to overcome as the social issues such as the negative perception or public and professional resistance against the adoption of AI. Therefore, there must be an effort to educate both clinicians and public about the nature of AI and its practical applications (Reddy & Cooper, 2021).

SUMMARY

- The emergence of Big Data has necessitated the need for advanced analytical techniques like AI
- AI replicates aspects of human intelligence and is capable of autonomous learning
- There are several categories of AI of which machine learning is the most popular approach
- AI is being applied in many disciplines, including medicine

REVIEW QUESTIONS

- Does the term 'Artificial Intelligence' adequately describe the description and nature of AI models?
- Consider the categorization of AI in this chapter. Does it match the available and current use of AI?
- There are only a few studies that validate the efficacy of AI in healthcare in terms of improvement in administrative or clinical outcomes. Why is this the case?
- What steps do you think have to be taken to enable the wider adoption and integration of AI in healthcare?
- Would there be autonomous 'AI clinicians' replacing human clinicians in the future?

References

Adlung, L., Cohen, Y., Mor, U., & Elinav, E. (2021). Machine learning in clinical decision making. *Med, 2*(6), 642–665. https://doi.org/10.1016/j.medj.2021.04.006

Agrawal, M., Hegselmann, S., Lang, H., Kim, Y., & Sontag, D. (2022). Large language models are zero-shot clinical information extractors. *arXiv preprint arXiv:2205.12689.*

Aung, Y. Y. M., Wong, D. C. S., & Ting, D. S. W. (2021). The promise of artificial intelligence: A review of the opportunities and challenges of artificial intelligence in healthcare. *Br Med Bull, 139*(1), 4–15. https://doi.org/10.1093/bmb/ldab016

Baclic, O., Tunis, M., Young, K., Doan, C., Swerdfeger, H., & Schonfeld, J. (2020). Challenges and opportunities for public health made possible by advances in natural language processing. *Can Commun Dis Rep, 46*(6), 161–168. https://doi.org/10.14745/ccdr.v46i06a02

Bajwa, J., Munir, U., Nori, A., & Williams, B. (2021). Artificial intelligence in healthcare: Transforming the practice of medicine. *Future Healthc J, 8*(2), e188–e194. https://doi.org/10.7861/fhj.2021-0095

Bartneck, C., Lütge, C., Wagner, A., & Welsh, S. (2021a). *An introduction to ethics in robotics and AI.* https://doi.org/10.1007/978-3-030-51110-4

Bartneck, C., Lütge, C., Wagner, A., & Welsh, S. (2021b). What Is AI? In *An introduction to ethics in robotics and AI* (pp. 5–16). https://doi.org/10.1007/978-3-030-51110-4_2

Bengio, Y., Lecun, Y., & Hinton, G. (2021). Deep learning for AI. *Commun ACM, 64*(7), 58–65. https://doi.org/10.1145/3448250

Bi, Q., Goodman, K.E., Kaminsky, J., & Lessler, J. (2019). What is machine learning? A primer for the epidemiologist. *Am J Epidemiol, 188*(12), 2222–2239. https://doi.org/10.1093/aje/kwz189

Butz, M. (2021). Towards strong AI. *KI - Künstliche Intelligenz, 35.* https://doi.org/10.1007/s13218-021-00705-x

Cappa, F., Oriani, R., Peruffo, E., & McCarthy, I. (2021). Big data for creating and capturing value in the digitalized environment: Unpacking the effects of volume, variety, and veracity on firm performance*. *J Prod Innov Manag, 38*(1), 49–67. https://doi.org/10.1111/jpim.12545

Chen, J. S., & Baxter, S. L. (2022). Applications of natural language processing in ophthalmology: Present and future. *Front Med (Lausanne), 9,* 906554. https://doi.org/10.3389/fmed.2022.906554

Cuzzolin, F., Morelli, A., Cîrstea, B., & Sahakian, B. J. (2020). Knowing me, knowing you: Theory of mind in AI. *Psychol Med, 50*(7), 1057–1061. https://doi.org/10.1017/s0033291720000835

Desai, A. N. (2020). Artificial intelligence: Promise, pitfalls, and perspective. *JAMA, 323*(24), 2448–2449. https://doi.org/10.1001/jama.2020.8737

Fjelland, R. (2020). Why general artificial intelligence will not be realized. *Humanities and Social Sciences Communications, 7*(10). https://doi.org/10.1057/s41599-020-0494-4

Ganguli, I., Gordon William, J., Lupo, C., Sands-Lincoln, M., George, J., Jackson, G., Rhee, K., & Bates David, W. Machine learning and the pursuit of high-value health care. *NEJM Catalyst, 1*(6). https://doi.org/10.1056/CAT.20.0094

GAO. (2020). *Artificial Intelligence in Health Care.* U. S. G. A. Office.

Gilson, A., Safranek, C. W., Huang, T., Socrates, V., Chi, L., Taylor, R. A., & Chartash, D. (2023). How does ChatGPT perform on the United States medical licensing examination? The implications of large language models for medical education and knowledge assessment. *JMIR Med Educ, 9,* e45312. https://doi.org/10.2196/45312

Gruetzemacher, R., & Paradice, D. (2022). Deep transfer learning & beyond: Transformer language models in information systems research. *ACM Comput Surv, 54*(10s), 1–35. https://doi.org/10.1145/3505245

Heidrich-Meisner, V., Lauer, M., Igel, C., & Riedmiller, M. (2007). Reinforcement learning in a Nutshell. in ESANN 2007: 15th European Symposium on Artificial Neural Networks, ES2007-4, D-side Publications, pp. 277–288, 15th European Symposium on Artificial Neural Networks, Brügge, Belgium, 25/04/2007. https://www.elen.ucl.ac.be/Proceedings/esann/esannpdf/es2007-4.pdf

Hintze, A. (2016). Understanding the four types of AI, from reactive robots to self-aware beings. *The Conversation.* Retrieved 30th June 2022 from https://theconversation.com/understanding-the-four-types-of-ai-from-reactive-robots-to-self-aware-beings-67616

Ingrand, F., & Ghallab, M. (2017). Deliberation for autonomous robots: A survey. *Artificial Intelligence.* https://doi.org/0.1016/j.artint.2014.11.003

Jordan, M. I., Mithcell, T. M. (2015). Machine learning: Trends, perspectives, and prospects. *Science, 349*(6245), 255–260.

Józefowicz, R., Vinyals, O., Schuster, M., Shazeer, N. M., & Wu, Y. (2016). Exploring the limits of language modeling. *ArXiv, abs/1602.02410.*

LeCun, Y., Bengio, Y., & Hinton, G. (2015). Deep learning. *Nature, 521*(7553), 436–444. https://doi.org/10.1038/nature14539

Lidströmer, N., Aresu, F., & Ashrafian, H. (2021). Basic concepts of artificial intelligence: Primed for clinicians. In Niklas Lidströmer, Federica Aresu, & Hutan Ashrafian (Eds.), *Artificial intelligence* (pp. 1–19). https://doi.org/10.1007/978-3-030-58080-3_1-1

Liebrenz, M., Schleifer, R., Buadze, A., Bhugra, D., & Smith, A. (2023). Generating scholarly content with ChatGPT: Ethical challenges for medical publishing. *Lancet Digit Health.* https://doi.org/10.1016/S2589-7500(23)00019-5

Litman, M. et al. (2021). Gathering Strength, Gathering Storms: The One Hundred Year Study on Artificial Intelligence (AI100) 2021 Study Panel Report. Stanford University, Stanford, CA, September 2021. Doc: http://ai100.stanford.edu/2021-report. Accessed: September 16, 2021.

Luitse, D., & Denkena, W. (2021). The great transformer: Examining the role of large language models in the political economy of AI. *Big Data Soc, 8*(2), 20539517211047734. https://doi.org/10.1177/20539517211047734

Madai, V., & Higgins, D. (2021). Artificial intelligence in healthcare: Lost in translation? ArXiv, abs/2107.13454

Montagnon, E., Cerny, M., Cadrin-Chenevert, A., Hamilton, V., Derennes, T., Ilinca, A., Vandenbroucke-Menu, F., Turcotte, S., Kadoury, S., & Tang, A. (2020). Deep learning workflow in radiology: A primer. *Insights Imaging, 11*(1), 22. https://doi.org/10.1186/s13244-019-0832-5

Patel, S. B., & Lam, K. (2023). ChatGPT: The future of discharge summaries? *Lancet Digit Health.* https://doi.org/10.1016/S2589-7500(23)00021-3

Reddy, S. (2018). Use of artificial intelligence in healthcare delivery. In T. F. Heston (Ed.), *Ehealth-making health care smarter.* Intech Open. https://doi.org/10.5772/intechopen.74714

Reddy, S. (2020a). Artificial intelligence and healthcare—why they need each other? *J Hosp Manag Health Policy, 5.* https://jhmhp.amegroups.com/article/view/6455

Reddy, S., Allan, S., Coghlan, S., & Cooper, P. (2020). A governance model for the application of AI in health care. *J Am Med Inform Assoc, 27*(3), 491–497. https://doi.org/10.1093/jamia/ocz192

Reddy, S., & Cooper, P. (2021). Health workforce learning in response to artificial intelligence. In K. Butler-Henderson, K. Day, & K. Gray (Eds.), *The health information workforce: Current and future developments* (pp. 129–137). Springer International Publishing. https://doi.org/10.1007/978-3-030-81850-0_8

Reddy, S., Fox, J., & Purohit, M. P. (2019). Artificial intelligence-enabled healthcare delivery. *J R Soc Med, 112*(1), 22–28. https://doi.org/10.1177/0141076818815510

Reddy, S., Rogers, W., Makinen, V. P., Coiera, E., Brown, P., Wenzel, M., Weicken, E., Ansari, S., Mathur, P., Casey, A., & Kelly, B. (2021). Evaluation framework to guide implementation of AI systems into healthcare settings. *BMJ Health Care Inform, 28*(1). https://doi.org/10.1136/bmjhci-2021-100444

Tan, H. (2017). A brief history and technical review of the expert system research. *IOP Conf Ser: Mater Sci Eng, 242,* 012111. https://doi.org/10.1088/1757-899x/242/1/012111

The Lancet Digital. (2023). ChatGPT: Friend or foe? *Lancet Digit Health.* https://doi.org/10.1016/S2589-7500(23)00023-7

Vaswani, A., Shazeer, N., Parmar, N., Uszkoreit, J., Jones, L., Gomez, A., Kaiser, L., & Polosukhin, I. (2017). Attention is all you need. NIPS.

Yamashita, R., Nishio, M., Do, R. K. G., & Togashi, K. (2018). Convolutional neural networks: An overview and application in radiology. *Insights Imaging, 9*(4), 611–629. https://doi.org/10.1007/s13244-018-0639-9

Yang, X., Chen, A., PourNejatian, N., Shin, H. C., Smith, K. E., Parisien, C., Compas, C., Martin, C., Costa, A. B., Flores, M. G., Zhang, Y., Magoc, T., Harle, C. A., Lipori, G., Mitchell, D. A., Hogan, W. R., Shenkman, E. A., Bian, J., & Wu, Y. (2022). A large language model for electronic health records. *NPJ Digit Med, 5*(1), 194. https://doi.org/10.1038/s41746-022-00742-2

Yao, X., Rushlow, D. R., Inselman, J. W., McCoy, R. G., Thacher, T. D., Behnken, E. M., Bernard, M. E., Rosas, S. L., Akfaly, A., Misra, A., Molling, P. E., Krien, J. S., Foss, R. M., Barry, B. A., Siontis, K. C., Kapa, S., Pellikka, P. A., Lopez-Jimenez, F., Attia, Z. I., … Noseworthy, P. A. (2021). Artificial intelligence-enabled electrocardiograms for identification of patients with low ejection fraction: A pragmatic, randomized clinical trial. *Nat Med, 27*(5), 815–819. https://doi.org/10.1038/s41591-021-01335-4

Zhang, D. et al. (2021). *Artificial intelligence index report 2021.* Stanford University.

Further Reading

Reddy, S. (2020b). *Artificial intelligence: Applications in healthcare delivery* (1st ed.). Productivity Press. https://doi.org/10.4324/9780429317415

Russell, Stuart J. (2010). *Artificial intelligence: A modern approach.* Prentice Hall.

Scott, I. A. (2021). Demystifying machine learning: A primer for physicians. *Intern Med J, 51*(9), 1388–1400. https://doi.org/10.1111/imj.15200

Zhang, D. et al. (2022). The AI Index 2022 Annual Report. AI Index Steering Committee, Stanford Institute for Human-Centered AI, Stanford University.

2

Applications of AI in Healthcare

Joe Zhang
Imperial College London, London, UK

Stephen Whebell
Townsville Hospital, Townsville, Australia

LEARNING OBJECTIVES

- Discuss the importance of healthcare data in relation to Artificial Intelligence.
- Identify areas and mechanisms that AI is being applied in healthcare, including:
  1. Important algorithms and use cases in computer vision AI
  2. Different approaches and risks of clinical decision support AI in electronic health records
  3. Emerging use cases for natural language processing AI
- Describe how artificial intelligence bias can widen healthcare disparity.

Introduction

The past decade has seen an exponential growth in interest, research, and investment into clinical applications of Artificial Intelligence (AI) (Zhang, Whebell, et al., 2022). While the early promise of wholesale transformation in how we deliver healthcare has not been achieved, our understanding of AI as a whole has matured, and we have also obtained an appreciation of how AI is best positioned within the healthcare space for the greatest effect (Rajpurkar et al., 2022). Rather than a revolution, we are now experiencing an evolution; and rather than AI-centred transformation, we are learning how to use AI selectively, to improve efficiency, safety, and diagnostic accuracy in particular areas of clinical need.

While algorithmic AI capabilities continue to advance, our use of AI in healthcare is limited by a reliance on medical data and an inability to generalize outside of its training (Topol, 2019). As discussed previously, the term 'Artificial Intelligence' belies the fact that we are very far from achieving a general machine intelligence. As such, our current systems can only give the *appearance* of intelligence, and often barely that.

DOI: 10.1201/9781003262152-2

Most AI systems in healthcare are developed using 'supervised learning' (Chapter 1) and perform a common type of task – which is to determine an outcome (from a set of known outcome labels) that is most strongly associated with a given set of data points. Such associations are learnt from a training process, where an algorithm is presented with data that is matched to outcome labels. For example, a self-driving car, trained on millions of hours of footage, can be taught to associate any image of a pedestrian crossing the street with labels such as 'danger' and 'braking'. As a result, if it sees new, live, video in the future with a pedestrian front and centre, it can predict 'danger' and 'braking' by association, with a high rate of accuracy. Substitute driving footage with any type of clinical data, and these associations with some pertinent clinical outcome, and this process is broadly accurate for many types of healthcare AI. Clinical data are numerous and detailed, and healthcare AI has the potential to be used in an almost unlimited number of clinical pathways. However, healthcare AI is also not a magical or general solution to clinical problems, and possesses many points that are vulnerable to failure (Panch et al., 2019).

Real-world applications have thus met with varying degrees of success and impact. The success of AI is highly context-dependent, and later chapters will discuss the host of ancillary infrastructural, clinical, and personnel-related challenges inherent in successful AI deployment. In this chapter, we will firstly discuss important considerations of AI models and data that are central to successful healthcare AI applications. We then look at specific fields where healthcare AI is at the cutting edge of practical application, including computer vision and radiomics, clinical decision support, and natural language processing.

A Brief Primer on Healthcare AI Models, Data, and Causality

Prior to discussing focused applications, it is important to establish some basics of healthcare AI development, models, and limitations. The novelty of AI is derived from both the ability to model new and unknown associations in data (rather than testing fit of data to a known model, as in traditional statistics), and the computational complexity of AI algorithms that allow the discovery of complex and hidden associations in big health data that may be otherwise uninterpretable to a clinician (Bzdok et al., 2018). As discussed in Chapter 1, supervised methods (the dominant type of AI used in clinical deployment) seek to create a set of computations that represent an association between data and an outcome. To do this, AI algorithms follow an iterative approach that tests different computations for transforming a dataset to produce the labelled outcomes most closely. This training process selects the most successful computations, which then become known as the AI model. Models can then be tested on separate data with known outcomes to assess accuracy, before being applied to new data (for which the predicted outcome is unknown) in a real-world deployment (Figure 2.1).

Beyond this broad description of method, the world of healthcare AI is entirely heterogeneous. Different AI algorithms exist which can be used to discover associations using differing mathematical strategies. These algorithms have defining characteristics such as computational requirements, performance on different data types, or suitability for

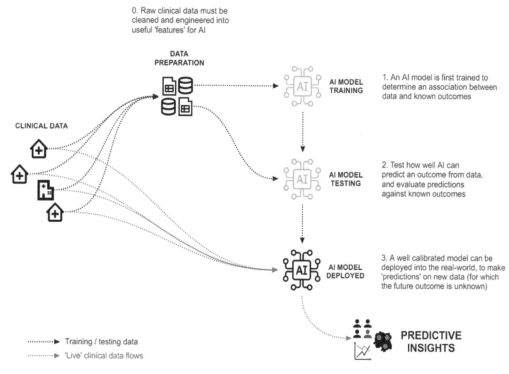

FIGURE 2.1

Training, testing, and deploying healthcare AI.

(Source: Authors.)

vast and complex datasets (Table 2.1). AI models may range from simple and transparent (showing a user what variables are most important for informing the prediction), to complex and impossible to interpret (a 'black box') (Reddy, 2022).

Perhaps more important than the algorithms are the data being used to train models (also known as 'features'). A key take-away of this chapter is that AI can only ever be as good as the data it was trained on. An AI algorithm cannot think, it cannot intelligently extrapolate, and it cannot deduce. It can only demonstrate an association based on the data and labels that it is provided. Therefore, poor-quality data, insufficient data, and inaccurate outcome labels used for training are all among the most important contributors to AI failures (Whang et al., 2021). 'Out-of-dataset' scenarios are common in the real world, and can result in adverse consequences from attempting to predict using new information that the model has not seen before, or predicting incorrect information on data the model has previously learnt to associate with an inaccurate outcome (Zhang, Budhdeo, et al., 2022). In our self-driving car scenario, these are respectively akin to experiencing a combination of scenarios that the AI has never seen before, thus confusing it in terms of what outputs to offer, and seeing an object or illusion that looks similar to pedestrian but is not, and therefore causing an incorrect output to 'brake'.

Even vast data of high completeness is not a panacea, as most routinely available healthcare data reflects bias in healthcare provision (Norori et al., 2021). For example,

TABLE 2.1

Supervised Learning Algorithms for Training Predictive Healthcare AI Models on Clinical Datasets

Algorithm	Description
Linear regression	Common machine learning algorithm used to understand the relationship between multiple dependent variables, and a continuous independent variable. A relationship is discovered by plotting a line of best fit between variables that minimizes the distance of variables from the line. Used in observational research to 'explain' relationships, as well as in prediction. Popular for simple, tabular clinical data.
Logistic regression	Similar to linear regression, but outputs are categorical (e.g., whether an event takes place, or not). Uses a logistic or sigmoid function that fits values to "0" or "1". Popular for simple, tabular clinical data.
Support vector machine	Classes of data are separated using a 'hyperplane', which is a boundary that maintains maximal separation between points in each class. A hyperplane is a boundary in n-dimensional space (corresponding to the number of features). Effective for clinical data where there is a strong and plausible separation between classes that is likely to be represented in the data, and where there are numerous dimensions. Typically applied to tabular and imaging data.
Random Forest	Uses an algorithmic technique based on 'decision trees', where classification is abstracted into a series of decisions and branches, matched to consequences. A random forest constructs multiple explanatory trees for each data and merges them to improve accuracy. Good explainability, due to ability to view sequence of decisions leading to classification output. Efficient handling for large tabular datasets.
XGBoost	A state-of-the-art tree-based algorithm that makes use of 'gradient boosting'. Rather than merging many decision trees (as in Random Forest), XGBoost will build new trees to compensate for inaccurate predictions in previous trees. XGBoost is currently the optimal algorithm for tabular datasets and outperforms deep learning in most instances.
Neural network	Discussed in *Chapter 1 – deep learning*. In the healthcare domain, neural networks can process highly complex associations. Networks incorporate many individual 'nodes' that each take an input, conduct a transformation, and 'fire' an output to a neighbouring node if a threshold is reached. Like synaptic networks in the brain, neural networks can replicate complex associations through weighted 'firing' patterns. Neural networks are the basis for all advanced healthcare AI applications on complex, multi-modal, and time-series data, including in computer vision and natural language processing.
Reinforcement learning	This is an emerging and powerful approach for training model prediction behaviours. By representing a patient's medical trajectory as a series of states, decisions ("actions") and subsequent positive or negative events, reinforcement learning (RL) approaches can train a model to select certain actions by computationally rewarding decisions that lead to positive events, and disincentivising those leading to negative events. RL is particularly reliant on data, sample size, and computational power.

consider a healthcare service where a minority demographic has little interaction with primary care doctors (perhaps for reasons of socioeconomic circumstance and racial bias). As a result, more individuals are not referred to a specialty service even when referral is needed. This is reflected in recorded healthcare data as low rates of referral for this minority. However, in training an AI model to predict *need for referral*, an algorithm will interpret these low rates of referral as *lack of need for referral*, with a strong association to the minority demographic. As a result, in deployment, the model will predict 'no referral' for patients of this demographic even when warranted, thus exacerbating existing encoded biases. This is not a hypothetical scenario – AI models deployed in the USA for predicting crime based on incarceration data, may positively identify most black residents (McKay, 2020). Similarly, models deployed by companies for selecting ideal candidates for executive job positions would always prefer to identify white, male, candidates (Tilmes, 2022). Without high quality, unbiased data, artificial intelligence becomes "artificial stupidity".

Finally, it is essential to appreciate that AI models (no matter how complex) have no direct relationship to causality. While there is a particular tendency for clinicians to apply a causal way of thinking to AI model outputs ("the models says that the patient is going to arrest because of this laboratory and physiological data"), this is a fallacy, as models are not trained under a causal framework, and can only be trained on data for events that occurred (without a counterfactual) (The INFORM-lab et al., 2019). As a result, the rules and associations embedded within a model are not a representation of real-world biological or pathological pathways that cause outcomes. This is important because subtle changes in input data (for example – as a result of population shifts, or data acquisition practices) mean that particular associations in the model may no longer hold true. The solution to this is monitoring of the model in deployment, and re-validation.

Despite these caveats, AI remains a powerful tool. Great strides in algorithmic complexity and in our ability to leverage multi-modal healthcare data have made it possible to develop transformational use cases across different healthcare domains, which we will discuss in the following sections.

Computer Vision and Medical Images

Computer vision is arguably the most successful domain of artificial intelligence, both in healthcare, and more generally. We see this in everyday life, with tasks such as automated labelling of online photo albums with known faces and pets or more simple tasks such as number plate recognition on toll roads. In healthcare, the interpretation of visual information is essential – from diagnosis of skin lesions to interpretation of four-dimensional (space and time) MRI sequences. This success is most prominent with the use of radiological or diagnostic medical imaging data (radiomics); as demonstrated by academic research output, real-world validation and regulatory device approvals. However, almost any visual data is accessible to AI algorithms, including (but not limited to): clinical or patient provided photographs and videos, digital microscopy and histology, digital fundoscopy, optical coherence tomography and endoscopically or laparoscopically derived images.

How Computers See – Images to Numbers to Meaning

A digital image is fundamentally an array composed of individual pixels. Each pixel contains information about its position in the image and its intensity or brightness. In grayscale (black and white) images each pixel contains a number that represents its appearance between completely white and completely black (Figure 2.2). In colour images, there are separate arrays or channels for red, green and blue (for RGB encoding).

Images are Numbers

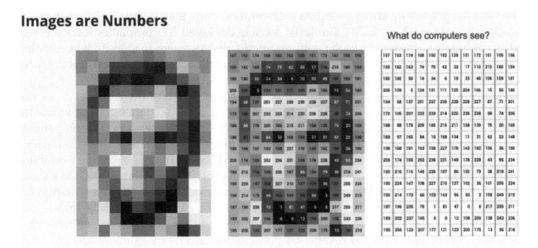

An Image is a matrix of numbers ranging between 0 and 255 across R/G/B color channels.

FIGURE 2.2
Image conversion to numbers.

(Credit: Golan Levin.)

While the final visual representation of the image is displayed, the underlying array of numbers provides a structured array of data that may be utilized in a variety of algorithms. The complexity of this data is increased for videos (a series of images) and for images that contain three-dimensional or spatial data such as computed tomography (CT) or magnetic resonance (MR) images. CT and MR images are composed of voxels, the 3D equivalent of pixels. Voxel size varies depending on the way in which the images were acquired and processed, but ultimately contains similar information to pixels regarding their position in the image and its intensity.

Deriving meaning from these complex data structures can appear daunting; however, utility has been demonstrated from a wide array for computational and algorithmic approaches. These range from unsupervised clustering to generate groups of similar images to computationally expensive and complex deep neural networks for image classification, segmentation, transformation and even generation.

The use of deep learning, specifically convolutional neural networks (CNNs), has dominated recent advances in computer vision (Yamashita et al., 2018). This is primarily due to demonstrated performance in both real-world and benchmarking datasets (Russakovsky et al., 2015), relative computational efficiency via inherent dimensionality reduction and robustness to messy input data with limited image pre-processing requirement. These advantages are largely due to the specific architecture of CNNs (see Chapter 1), which is inspired by neuron connectivity within an animal visual cortex. In the visual cortex, individual neurons respond only to specific areas of the visual field, overlapping to cumulatively cover the entire visual field. In a CNN an image is inputted as a tensor with a known shape – height (in pixels) x width (in pixels) x channels (one for grayscale, three for RGB, potentially more for multi-dimensional images). A kernel or filter of a substantially smaller size than the whole image (e.g., 5 x 5 pixels) is then applied in an overlapping manner across the entire image. The filter output (or convolution) results in the generation of a feature for an area of pixels, rather than for each individual pixel or the image as a whole. This enables the representation and recognition of small details across the image. The features generated by this process are represented as a feature map of reduced dimensions to the original image. This feature map then undergoes a pooling process where the spatial size is further reduced. This process of convolution and pooling may be repeated several times, enabling the identification of dominant features within the image and increasing computational efficiency through dimensionality reduction. Finally, the output of this process is fed to a fully connected neural network and ultimately to an output layer where the desired task is completed.

A significant downside of CNN use for visual medical data is the need for high-volume accurately labelled training data. While relatively computationally efficient, due to the use of small details within images as features, many examples are required to train most examples of a CNN to perform well. CNNs are also a prime example of deep learning as a "black box" – it is very difficult to tell what an algorithm has used to reach the conclusion presented at its output. This problem is particularly pertinent in healthcare, where the eventual use of "black box" models will be in patient care.

Radiomics

Modern healthcare is dependent on radiological imaging to facilitate accurate diagnosis of pathology, track the progress of disease and facilitate procedures. The data associated with radiological medical imaging is called radiomics. Typical imaging modalities from which radiomics are generated include X-ray (XR), computerized tomography (CT) scanning, ultrasound (US) and magnetic resonance imaging (MRI).

The demand for radiological imaging and its expert interpretation by radiologists is high, with some tertiary centres performing and interpreting over 1000 studies per day (Côté & Smith, 2018). This significant volume of utilization makes radiomics an ideal use case for artificial intelligence – to offload and assist specialist radiologists or provide near-expert interpretation in areas where there is no specialist available. Training data is plentiful and well labelled due to routine interpretation and reporting by experts. Training data also follows a consistent format and structure with standardized methods of image acquisition and storage. This is due to the Digital Imaging and Communications in Medicine (DICOM) standard. Furthermore, this data is stored in a self-contained, well-organized system that is designed for secure storage and rapid retrieval of both images and reporting data – known as a picture archiving and communication system (PACS). The combination of these factors has bolstered radiomic use in AI, resulting in its widespread use in research and increasingly in the real world.

Disease diagnosis and disease detection are the most common tasks undertaken by AI using radiomic data. Most applications in this domain have a relatively narrow focus, such as classifying lung nodules on CT scans as benign or cancerous with performance as good or better than expert classification. A narrow focus does not necessarily preclude complexity of data or analysis – AI has also seen considerable use in MR sequences of the whole brain to differentiate normal age-related changes from changes associated with cognitive impairment and Alzheimer's disease (Frizzell et al., 2022). "General purpose" image interpretation has also been explored, with fully automated reporting of chest XR images across a diverse range of specialties demonstrating improved accuracy across multiple clinical findings (Seah et al., 2021).

Automated quantification of findings and image segmentation to support human interpretation of radiology is another notable use of AI in radiomics. Most radiology derived severity grading systems involve measurement of structures and findings. Via identification of relevant structures and quantification of abnormalities, AI has the potential to improve the efficiency of radiologists' interpretation of complex images. Cardiac MRI is one such field where AI has great potential in this regard. Cardiac MRI involves the acquisition of 4D (3D + time) images of a beating heart. Interpretation requires labour-intensive image reconstruction, labelling and measurement of the cardiac chambers, cardiac muscle, valves and even blood flow throughout a heartbeat. Within this process, there exists both intra- and inter-observer variability and differing methodologies that can result in inconsistent interpretation. Automatic segmentation and measurement of the cardiac chambers using deep convolutional neural networks has been shown to be more consistent and time-efficient than standard manual or alternate algorithmic approaches (Fotaki et al., 2022). Similar approaches (with a variety of imaging modalities) have also been used for automated segmentation and measurement of lobes of the brain, measurement of brain herniation in response to injury, segmentation of lung lobes and the abdominal viscera.

Beyond disease diagnosis, disease detection and interpretation aids there are increasingly novel applications of AI in radiomics. Image acquisition may be improved via the use of AI – such as de-noising MR images or removing movement artefact from high-resolution CT images. AI may be able to derive novel radiomic biomarkers that can be used to predict the course of disease or chance of survival at varying intervals – this has been investigated in situations such as CT images of pulmonary fibrosis, MR images of the heart and chest XR images of acute respiratory distress syndrome (ARDS). AI can also aid in the use of portable, bedside ultrasonography – both in live image interpretation as well as guiding inexperienced operators on how to position probes to acquire the best images (Voelker, 2020). Finally, generative AI models can be used to produce realistic synthetic medical images that have never existed previously. This has particular use for the augmentation of training data in model generation.

Photography, Videography, and Other Medical Images

Outside the well-contained, well-labelled and voluminous world of radiomics there is still a huge amount of digital visual medical data. This can include images captured by patients at home using smartphones, images and videos obtained during endoscopic procedures, clinical images and videos taken by clinicians, histological images from digital microscopy, retinal images and optical coherence tomography (Hormel et al., 2021). Automatic diagnosis of skin lesions based on smartphone photography by patients has been a particular area of success – with evaluation performance on part with dermatologists (Esteva et al., 2017). Videos taken of patients walking can be used for automated gait analysis – an important component of diagnosis of many neurological diseases and a useful tool in the rehabilitation setting (Sipari et al., 2022). Computational pathology and histology utilising AI is a field growing at an accelerating rate – with a wealth of data and labelling similar to radiomics (Cui & Zhang, 2021).

AI Computer Vision in the Real World – A Murkier Picture

Most published data in this field is retrospective, with limited validation in the real world (Kelly et al., 2022). Despite this, suites of software by commercial entities are already available utilising AI-assisted diagnostics using radiomics. The commercial availability of these tools is likely to continue to expand, with AI devices utilising radiomic data forming the bulk of recent regulatory approvals (Muehlematter et al., 2021). As discussed elsewhere, robust prospective validation and evaluation for bias is paramount for the successful use of AI in the real world. This is particularly true for AI models utilising imaging data, where while training and testing may be relatively self-contained, they may not reflect the real-world workflow where the models are ultimately deployed (see Case Study 1). Finally, bias within models has the potential to reflect clinician and system biases in patient care. A study recently demonstrated that an AI model was able to accurately predict patient self-reported race from XR data where clinicians cannot (Gichoya et al., 2022), even after attempts to degrade image quality and add noise. The implications of these findings are enormous – further raising the alarm on the absolute importance of evaluating bias within AI and model interpretability (understanding the "black box").

CASE STUDY 1   GOOGLE HEALTH DIABETIC RETINOPATHY FIELD TEST

Google Health is the health technology and AI branch of the Silicon Valley technology giant. The company has prioritized attempts at bringing health AI to low-resource and developing environments.

Diabetic retinopathy screening is a population health screening task that involves looking at retinal images (either through an ophthalmoscope or using pre-taken retinal photographs) and grading the extent of diabetic eye disease. Such diabetic complications can cause irreversible vision loss, and signs of diabetic disease in the eyes also indicate multi-organ complications elsewhere (such as in coronary arteries, or in the kidneys). Screening can help detect early signs of disease and indicate need for closer diabetic control and follow-up. The burden of such late-stage disease is particularly great in developing countries, where there is higher disease prevalence, coupled with a lack of resources to target interventions at the right population. Both resources for intervention, and resources for screening, are limited – thus, there is a great need to stratify the population and divert treatment to the groups that need it most.

This is a great opportunity for an AI application (Grzybowski et al., 2020) – increasing both access, and promoting cost savings (Dismuke, 2020). Google Health funded research for a model that could screen for retinopathy using automated analysis of retinal photos. In a landmark study, using deep learning computer vision algorithms, a model was developed on more than 128,000 images, and validated on 10,000 images, showing more than 90% accuracy in diagnosis tasks (Gulshan et al., 2016). The model further showed promising performance in evaluating photos against U.S. board-certified ophthalmologists (Krause et al., 2018).

Finally, the model was taken to a low-resource setting in Thailand (Beede et al., 2020). Despite promising performance in the 'lab', when tested in the real world, performance was found to fall far short of standards expected for diagnostic accuracy, workflow improvements, and patient experience. The authors made several key findings: (1) there was significant variation on how nurses captured retinal photographs, how workflows were modified to incorporate AI, and how results were taken onwards for referral; (2) there were significant resource disparities between clinical regions, and only two sites had a dedicated screening room where high-quality fundus photos could be taken; (3) real-world image quality overall was far poorer than the images used to train the model, containing local 'out-of-dataset' features such as a blurred areas, dark areas, and other quality problems that caused the model to reject many images; (4) the model relied on first world technological infrastructure, and slow hardware and network connectivity meant the overall pipeline was far more prone to failure and poor user-experience; (5) finally, even at optimal accuracy, model outputs were still considered a risk for missing cases, or false positives (necessitating an expensive an unnecessary hospital visit), discouraging patients from using the service.

As a case study, this is a very relevant illustration that healthcare applications rely on far more than algorithmic complexity. Real-world factors, including the quality and real-world representativeness of healthcare data, are the most important indicators of whether a model will succeed as an in-situ healthcare application.

EHR Clinical Decision Support

Imaging workflows are relatively self-contained, with models sending discrete predictive or diagnostic signals to be packaged up as a report for other clinicians. Outside of these workflows, the hospital environment is more complex, as decision-making is informed by a vast array of medical histories, symptoms, physiological observations, laboratory markers, clinical examination, investigation results, competing expert opinion, and often-intangible combinations of such factors that result in a holistic 'bedside view' of any patient. While AI would seem perfectly suited for such a complex environment, there are significant barriers which do not exist for computer vision use cases (Zhang, Mattie, et al., 2022). Even so, some of the most widely deployed healthcare AI applications operate in the electronic health record (EHR) clinical decision support (CDS) domain.

AI-Based Decision Support Applications

EHR data used in AI models is generally structured, carrying existing definitions of meaning (unstructured data will be discussed in the next section). EHR data is likely to use a medical coding language. These languages are dictionaries of categorical codes that represent different medical concepts (Benson & Grieve, 2016). International standards include the disease-focused International Statistical Classification of Diseases (ICD), and the more semantically rich SNOMED clinical terms (SNOMED-CT), which can use combinations of codes to represent most clinical interactions. While coding standardization is encouraged, and is key to integrating different data sources, many software suppliers may still use proprietary medical codes. Numerical test results and physiological values add an additional, valuable data source that can represent an overall view of a patient's history and current circumstance.

Within an inpatient setting, such data is frequently used in AI models for generating flags that predict significant clinical events. These models may be particularly useful in emergency decision-making situations where they can help clinicians triage and prioritize (hence, clinical "decision support"), or in situations where there may be case and information overload, and where at-risk patients may be missed – for example, where there is a high proportion of late sepsis diagnosis. In practice, due to the requirement to integrate such models into an EHR, many models are created and deployed by software suppliers. The *Epic* sepsis model is a prominent example, and has been deployed in hundreds of hospitals around the United States for flagging patients with likely sepsis for clinical attention and escalation (Wong et al., 2021). Other examples may include models which alert clinicians to patients at risk of deterioration or cardiac arrest, which make greater use of physiological trends and clinical assessment data (Romero-Brufau et al., 2021), often through predicting on a moving time window of data. In clinical deployment, these may be integrated in clinical monitoring hardware, or as a suite of tools for patient monitoring.

Outside of a hospital setting, AI can be applied to help decision-making in chronic disease management or in specialty referral. Much like a traditional risk score, identifying progression of diseases such as renal failure early can help undertake preventative measures, or early referral, or system optimization. One of the richest domains is the prediction of cardiovascular complications, where many traditional risk scores must now compete with AI alternatives for myocardial infarction and stroke risk (Cho et al., 2021). With the ability to integrate multi-centre or even regional data, there is potential to deploy decision support systems that inform population health interventions, through models for risk stratification or hospital load forecasting (Rea et al., 2019).

Algorithms for EHR Data

Such models may make use of algorithms such as XGBoost, which demonstrate advanced performance on tabular data (Shwartz-Ziv & Armon, 2021). In many cases, the additional complexity of deep learning results in only minimal performance gain over simpler algorithms, at the cost of heavy computational requirements, and also being a 'black box' for interpretation. Both of these negative trade-offs have significant real-world consequences. In short, monetary and computational cost of continual deployment of AI models must be considered in any development process, and an understanding of how models reach their conclusions is particularly vital in complex environments where clinicians must weigh up multiple extraneous data to inform treatment decisions.

However, a key consideration in these models is also the time-series component. While traditional algorithmic learning considers a table of cross-sectional information about a patient, it is important to appreciate that the pattern of patient characteristic change over time is a vital part of what defines subsequent outcomes (J. M. Lee & Hauskrecht, 2021). For example, a patient with low blood pressure is likely to experience a different outcome if their blood pressure has slowly dropped over the past few days, compared to a patient whose blood pressure has collapsed over 10 minutes. Considering how to engineer features that represent these longitudinal components or using deep learning models such as long short-term memory networks (LSTM) that can handle observations in a temporal sequence, are key to establishing useful real-world healthcare applications.

An additional strategy is to use agnostic data-driven techniques for identifying particular complex phenotypes of patients to support subsequent decision-making. These are unsupervised algorithms (Chapter 1) that can computationally discover distinct patient groups, defined by distinct characteristics. To be useful, phenotypes must be both clinically interpretable, and must make biological sense. Such algorithms may be less vulnerable to idiosyncrasies in clinical coding and outcome label quality, as they do not require prior outcome label definitions, or the restricted specification of features for training a supervised model. Basing decisions around certain phenotypes mimics a clinician-led decision-making process, where particular patterns of patient trajectory may be identified by a clinical team for association with need for a certain treatment. Validated phenotypes can be subsequently used as the predictor target in supervised models. While at a much earlier stage of implementation in practice, such approaches have been used in such use cases as guiding COVID-19 pandemic treatment pathways (Zhang et al., 2021), or in the identification of patient biological subgroups for anti-inflammatory treatment (Qin et al., 2022).

Dirty Data and Complex Environments

Compared to computer vision applications, there are additional barriers to success in clinical decision support. A primary barrier relates to dependency on routinely collected health record data and codes. In the primer section, we discussed broad problems with healthcare data, and this is most significant when trying to bring models from "bench to bedside" within EHRs (Whebell & Zhang, 2022). Where radiomics or signal-based models use data that is relatively objective (in that it is a consistently produced image or signal), routinely recorded codes are subject to quality issues from missing input, variable coding practices, clinician inaccuracy, and input biases. Important demographic data may be missing as there is less incentive (from reimbursements) to code these with high quality. These features often have great importance in predictive models. A further barrier is the previously mentioned complex environment that models are deployed in. The majority of information that clinicians use to make decisions is not available as computed data. Real-world treatments are guided to an extent by medical histories and quantitative values, but situational information from clinical examination, uncoded information, group consensus with an input of 'gut feeling' or 'clinical acumen' cannot yet be used to train a model. As such, models may underperform in the real world.

Overall, despite the widespread deployment of EHR CDS, real-world evaluations have largely shown underwhelming performance. The *Epic* sepsis model has been shown to greatly overpredict, ana also to miss considerable numbers of patients in practice (Habib et al., 2021). Similarly, deterioration prediction models may experience the same issues as crude non-AI scores, in over-prediction and false positive flags that result in clinician fatigue (Yu et al., 2021).

A Vital Component of a Healthcare Application

Regardless, the successful use of AI in the midst of vital and overloaded clinical pathways is an overwhelmingly important objective. While algorithmic science has progressed to remarkable levels, the ability to integrate and utilize existing data, to ensure consistent, high-quality and unbiased data, and to capture new useful data, lag behind. It is these areas that must be developed to ensure successful EHR CDS deployment into the future.

Natural Language Processing

An estimated 80% of healthcare data is unstructured free text, which means it is composed of narrative written speech, without further organization into tables or into a traditional database (Zhang, Symons, et al., 2022). Unlike coded medical data, which has clear definitions and structure that enable easy computation, unstructured data is more difficult to access and analyse. Despite this, huge amounts of informative data are contained within such narrative clinical notes, that go beyond the constraints of structured codes within electronic healthcare records (EHR).

Language, especially specialist medical language, is difficult for machines to interpret. This is because of diversity in content, a need for descriptive precision, and also in its semantic and syntactic complexity. Natural language processing (NLP) is a branch of AI that can effectively process words and sequences of words into a machine interpretable and analysable format. Unlike previous examples, we have explored that predict a real-world healthcare outcome, the AI in NLP is primarily used to generate a high-dimensional vector of numbers (or an 'embedding') that can numerically represent text, and which can then be used for subsequent computational tasks such as supervised prediction (Wu et al., 2020). It is important to distinguish the usage of NLP AI in creating such embeddings from the subsequent use of embeddings as features in separate AI models. Both stages are important in NLP healthcare applications.

Meaning from Text

The first attempts to represent language numerically did not utilize AI, but adopted measures such as counting the occurrence of words in a passage of text ('Bag of Words') (Qader et al., 2019). Any text passage can thus be represented by word frequency, which, while crude, serves for many real-world NLP based use cases outside of healthcare. For example, a model can be trained on counts of spam email words (labelled as 'spam') and counts of non-spam email words (labelled as 'not spam') for a simple spam filter.

One of the first usages of AI in the NLP embedding was the Word2vec algorithm (Mikolov et al., 2013), which used a neural network to capture contextual information about each unique word in a text. The neural network algorithm attempts to model the association between each word, and the words that surround it, thus capturing both semantic (meaning) and syntactic (structural) details. As discussed, this type of prediction produces an embedding, which can be considered as a long list of numbers that is usable for mathematical operations. Word2vec excels at capturing meaning. Famously, if you use embeddings in a mathematical operation to calculate "king - man + woman", you will receive the perfectly logical "queen" as an answer. This is because the embeddings that the model has learnt for "king" and "queen" capture semantic information about meanings such as "royalty", as well as their respective genders, by using context represented in words within surrounding text. Words with similar meanings and uses can be expected to have similar embeddings. As with the email spam example, one can use these embeddings (or a group of embeddings) as a feature in an AI model where meaning within text is important for prediction.

The most recent development in NLP embeddings has been the use of transformer models (Chapter 1) (Yang et al., 2020). Transformers also aim to encode text into a complex numerical representation but can learn such representations through tracking position and relationships of a text sequence, whilst processing and keeping memory of the entire passage of text (rather than a fixed window around the word of interest, as in Word2Vec). As such, words are encoded with reference to their context in *all* parts of a text passage. Transformer models are the basis of 'pre-trained' systems which have processed and subsequently hold memory of very large text inputs, such as the entirety of PubMed or Wikipedia. These models, such as BERT and GPT-3, hold an incredible degree of semantic and syntactic representation, and can be used to power highly realistic conversational AI, or further trained using selected relevant examples for specific healthcare applications.

NLP into Healthcare Utility

By training from large bodies of narrative EHR text or medical publications, NLP models can develop a deep contextual knowledge of medical concepts and syntactics. In practice, such models can be described in three categories of tasks: (1) information extraction – finding specific structured information from narrative free-text; (2) clinical prediction – using such extracted information, or using vectorized text embeddings, as a feature in prediction models; (3) workflow support – using the realistic language properties of large AI models for supporting clinical workflows.

During an information extraction task, an NLP model is used to identify and label information within narrative text, thus extracting terms into a structured format. Named entity recognition (NER) is the method most frequently seen in healthcare applications. Predefined categories (such as diseases, investigations, procedures etc) are the objective of classification tasks (Kundeti et al., 2016). An NLP model uses its understanding of meaning and context to locate and classify words or phrases into these categories. With more complex models, it is not necessary to have seen any particular word before. Instead, a category can be inferred by context, and a label can be inferred by similarity of embedding to other previously encountered sequences. Figure 2.3 shows how a model can label pertinent words in a medical narrative. The extraction of structured text has numerous healthcare applications. As discussed in the previous section, structured clinical coding is often inaccurate and incomplete. In healthcare systems where reimbursements are calculated using EHR clinical coding, there is great value in identifying missed information from text narratives. NER models may be used to identify pertinent codes that represent diseases, actions, and treatments that are reimbursable, and this service is a typical offering from large NLP platform companies (Bhatia et al., 2019). This same technique can

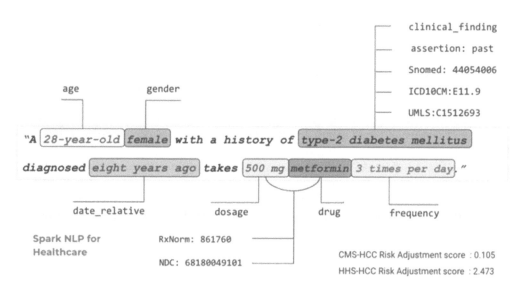

FIGURE 2.3
Labelling of key words in a medical narrative.

(Source: John Snow Labs.)

also greatly enrich the use of EHR data for medical research, both filling in event gaps in a patient's clinical coding record, but also including such data as demographic and social background information that generally exhibits poor coding quality. Such tasks may have previously fallen to teams of clinical expert manual annotators, but advanced NLP models have obvious advantages in cost and time. Increasingly, clinical trials have recognised the importance of NLP information extraction for tasks such as the identification of codes that might flag specific patients for trial recruitment (Idnay et al., 2021).

Structured or embedded meaning within narrative text can add feature richness to predictive signals. Extracted variables of importance, or chosen sequences embedded in vector format, can be input into supervised learning processes (possibly combining with other structured or multi-modal features), improving predictive performance in many circumstances. Particular examples of these include in psychiatric specialties, where narrative documentation may be particularly semantically rich. Descriptions of symptoms and trajectory have been used to predict suicide attempts (Tsui et al., 2021), predict disease and treatment outcomes, and diagnose disease progression or relapse (Lee et al., 2022). Numerous other similar use cases exist in other medical specialties (Gao et al., 2022), and have also been applied to big social media data for population health and infectious disease signalling (Conway et al., 2019). More advanced use cases include the deployment of near-real-time forecasting on signals from free text, such as for infectious disease signalling (Teo et al., 2021). The ability to predict on free text, as it is entered into the record, has advantages over traditional prediction models where laboratory markers and clinical codes may require time to achieve the level of completeness and quality required for an AI model to be performant.

Outside of healthcare, NLP can be used for streamlining processes and enriching interactions, through chatbots, translation services, and transcription services. With increasing recognition of clinician burnout from health information technology, and from the burden of minute documentation and administrative tasks, NLP is increasingly also recognised as a method for clinical workflow optimization. Strategies include improving quality of clinical notes from voice transcription (for example – *Amazon Transcribe Medical*), as well as turning longer narratives into more easily digestible summaries or writing narrative discharge summaries using the whole clinical admission record (Searle et al., 2022). We are currently seeing a newer generation of medically focused virtual patient assistants, which can help to triage and provide education to patients. However, concerns about AI safety and the propensity for verbose language outputs to 'hallucinate' incorrect information (Ji et al., 2022) mean that we are still some distance away from independent AI-conducted clinical consultations. This balance is no better illustrated than by the astonishing ability of large NLP models, such as "ChatGPT", to sustain realistic conversations, but occasionally provide wrong and potentially dangerous information. Finally, as generative models are used for creating synthetic medical images for training data, large language models may be fine-tuned to create synthetic text that preserves the meaning of clinical features but strips any identifying features to preserve privacy within narrative text (Ive, 2022).

Promising Future

In conclusion, NLP can be seen as one of the brightest frontiers of AI in medicine, due to the incredible power of large transformer models and the untapped potential of unstructured data. Like any AI, it is worth mentioning the substantial barriers to its successful application, which include infrastructure for data mining, where massive amounts of free text across multiple formats must be accessed and parsed. In addition, there is a relative sparsity of free text for training medicine-specific NLP models, in part due to concerns about patient privacy. While it is possible to strip identifiers from structured text, it is harder to do so in unstructured narratives, where there is a risk of models learning and subsequently utilising personal identifiable and sensitive information.

Conclusion

We stand in a moment of shifting sensibilities about AI applications in healthcare. For a decade, it has been easy to view healthcare AI as the future, greatly augmenting clinical capabilities and saving lives and resources. The truth is more complex, and real-world applications are littered with more failures than successes. In this chapter, we have discussed the landscape of healthcare AI applications from a more cautious lens that also considers its inherent limitations. We have considered how the AI model is only one part of a spectrum of considerations, and that it must be considered a tool that should be applied prudently and situationally (Higgins & Madai, 2020). We have highlighted exemplar healthcare AI fields that, through significant algorithmic and data advances, show great promise in active deployment.

Healthcare AI is, of course, not limited to the domains discussed. As wearables and patient-owned devices become more common, AI models that predict on personal data are becoming a key component in our daily lives. There is no better example than smart watches, which may utilize AI algorithms for adverse event and arrhythmia detection (Inui et al., 2020). Similarly, home monitoring devices and apps can now move traditional inpatient care to patients' homes, without requiring a clinician to be physically present. The increasing integration of multi-modal data such as genomics, move these fields from laboratory-based AI work in disease pathway and drug discovery, towards clinical applications, where objective genomic profiles are likely to transform personalized risk prediction and decision support (Acosta et al., 2022). Ultimately, it is likely that the greatest potential will come from combining multiple modalities of data and techniques together, assisted by advanced NLP applications that can interface directly and independently with patients.

We conclude this chapter by proposing that the future of health AI applications must focus on integration, quality, and bias in healthcare data (Andrew Ng, 2021), as well as the entire 'supply chain' of needs and requirements for an AI application to be successful in the real world (Zhang, Budhdeo, et al., 2022). These factors will be discussed in greater detail in the following chapters.

SUMMARY

- Healthcare AI is approaching an evolutionary stage that requires considered application to relevant use cases of high clinical value.
- AI is a modelling tool and has no independent intelligence outside of learning from the data it is trained on.
- Healthcare AI is only as good as the data used for training. Good-quality and unbiased healthcare data are key to successful application.
- Computer vision leads healthcare applications through advanced algorithmic techniques, high-quality standardized data, and well-defined clinical workflows.
- Electronic health record (HER) AI has great potential for alleviating and overloaded workflows but must consider barriers related to clinical environments and data quality.
- Natural language processing is a promising frontier for making use of huge quantities of untapped and rich healthcare data, for improving pathways and for clinical prediction.

REVIEW QUESTIONS

- What are potential determinants of AI application success outside of the AI algorithms themselves?
- How can we ensure the quality of healthcare data for AI uses?
- How can AI be used to reduce healthcare disparity, rather than widen it?
- What will the applied healthcare AI landscape look like in ten years' time?
- What does multi-modal personalized healthcare look like?

References

Acosta, J. N., Falcone, G. J., Rajpurkar, P., & Topol, E. J. (2022). Multimodal biomedical AI. *Nature Medicine, 28*(9), 1773–1784. https://doi.org/10.1038/s41591-022-01981-2

Andrew, Ng. (2021, June). *MLOps: From model-centric to data-centric AI*. https://www.deeplearning.ai/wp-content/uploads/2021/06/MLOps-From-Model-centric-to-Data-centric-AI.pdf

Beede, E., Baylor, E., Hersch, F., Iurchenko, A., Wilcox, L., Ruamviboonsuk, P., & Vardoulakis, L. M. (2020). A human-centered evaluation of a deep learning system deployed in clinics for the detection of diabetic retinopathy. *Proceedings of the 2020 CHI Conference on Human Factors in Computing Systems*, 1–12. https://doi.org/10.1145/3313831.3376718

Benson, T., & Grieve, G. (2016). *Principles of health interoperability: SNOMED CT, HL7 and FHIR*. Springer International Publishing. https://doi.org/10.1007/978-3-319-30370-3

Bhatia, P., Celikkaya, B., Khalilia, M., & Senthivel, S. (2019). Comprehend medical: A named entity recognition and relationship extraction web service. *2019 18th IEEE International Conference on Machine Learning and Applications (ICMLA)*, 1844–1851. https://doi.org/10.1109/ICMLA.2019.00297

Bzdok, D., Altman, N., & Krzywinski, M. (2018). Statistics versus machine learning. *Nature Methods, 15*(4), 233–234. https://doi.org/10.1038/nmeth.4642

Cho, S.-Y., Kim, S.-H., Kang, S.-H., Lee, K. J., Choi, D., Kang, S., Park, S. J., Kim, T., Yoon, C.-H., Youn, T.-J., & Chae, I.-H. (2021). Pre-existing and machine learning-based models for cardiovascular risk prediction. *Scientific Reports, 11*(1), 8886. https://doi.org/10.1038/s41598-021-88257-w

Conway, M., Hu, M., & Chapman, W. W. (2019). Recent advances in using natural language processing to address public health research questions using social media and consumer generated data. *Yearbook of Medical Informatics, 28*(01), 208–217. https://doi.org/10.1055/s-0039-1677918

Côté, M. J., & Smith, M. A. (2018). Forecasting the demand for radiology services. *Health Systems, 7*(2), 79–88. https://doi.org/10.1080/20476965.2017.1390056

Cui, M., & Zhang, D. Y. (2021). Artificial intelligence and computational pathology. *Laboratory Investigation, 101*(4), 412–422. https://doi.org/10.1038/s41374-020-00514-0

Dismuke, C. (2020). Progress in examining cost-effectiveness of AI in diabetic retinopathy screening. *The Lancet Digital Health, 2*(5), e212–e213. https://doi.org/10.1016/S2589-7500(20)30077-7

Esteva, A., Kuprel, B., Novoa, R. A., Ko, J., Swetter, S. M., Blau, H. M., & Thrun, S. (2017). Dermatologist-level classification of skin cancer with deep neural networks. *Nature, 542*(7639), 115–118. https://doi.org/10.1038/nature21056

Fotaki, A., Puyol-Antón, E., Chiribiri, A., Botnar, R., Pushparajah, K., & Prieto, C. (2022). Artificial intelligence in cardiac MRI: Is clinical adoption forthcoming? *Frontiers in Cardiovascular Medicine, 8*, 818765. https://doi.org/10.3389/fcvm.2021.818765

Frizzell, T. O., Glashutter, M., Liu, C. C., Zeng, A., Pan, D., Hajra, S. G., D'Arcy, R. C. N., & Song, X. (2022). Artificial intelligence in brain MRI analysis of Alzheimer's disease over the past 12 years: A systematic review. *Ageing Research Reviews, 77*, 101614. https://doi.org/10.1016/j.arr.2022.101614

Gao, Y., Dligach, D., Christensen, L., Tesch, S., Laffin, R., Xu, D., Miller, T., Uzuner, O., Churpek, M. M., & Afshar, M. (2022). A scoping review of publicly available language tasks in clinical natural language processing. *Journal of the American Medical Informatics Association, 29*(10), 1797–1806. https://doi.org/10.1093/jamia/ocac127

Gichoya, J. W., Banerjee, I., Bhimireddy, A. R., Burns, J. L., Celi, L. A., Chen, L.-C., Correa, R., Dullerud, N., Ghassemi, M., Huang, S.-C., Kuo, P.-C., Lungren, M. P., Palmer, L. J., Price, B. J., Purkayastha, S., Pyrros, A. T., Oakden-Rayner, L., Okechukwu, C., Seyyed-Kalantari, L., … Zhang, H. (2022). AI recognition of patient race in medical imaging: A modelling study. *The Lancet Digital Health, 4*(6), e406–e414. https://doi.org/10.1016/S2589-7500(22)00063-2

Grzybowski, A., Brona, P., Lim, G., Ruamviboonsuk, P., Tan, G. S. W., Abramoff, M., & Ting, D. S. W. (2020). Artificial intelligence for diabetic retinopathy screening: A review. *Eye, 34*(3), 451–460. https://doi.org/10.1038/s41433-019-0566-0

Gulshan, V., Peng, L., Coram, M., Stumpe, M. C., Wu, D., Narayanaswamy, A., Venugopalan, S., Widner, K., Madams, T., Cuadros, J., Kim, R., Raman, R., Nelson, P. C., Mega, J. L., & Webster, D. R. (2016). Development and validation of a deep learning algorithm for detection of diabetic retinopathy in retinal fundus photographs. *JAMA, 316*(22), 2402. https://doi.org/10.1001/jama.2016.17216

Habib, A. R., Lin, A. L., & Grant, R. W. (2021). The epic sepsis model falls short – The importance of external validation. *JAMA Internal Medicine, 181*(8), 1040. https://doi.org/10.1001/jamainternmed.2021.3333

Higgins, D., & Madai, V. I. (2020). From bit to bedside: A practical framework for artificial intelligence product development in healthcare. *Advanced Intelligent Systems, 2*(10), 2000052. https://doi.org/10.1002/aisy.202000052

Hormel, T. T., Hwang, T. S., Bailey, S. T., Wilson, D. J., Huang, D., & Jia, Y. (2021). Artificial intelligence in OCT angiography. *Progress in Retinal and Eye Research, 85*, 100965. https://doi.org/10.1016/j.preteyeres.2021.100965

Idnay, B., Dreisbach, C., Weng, C., & Schnall, R. (2021). A systematic review on natural language processing systems for eligibility prescreening in clinical research. *Journal of the American Medical Informatics Association, 29*(1), 197–206. https://doi.org/10.1093/jamia/ocab228

Inui, T., Kohno, H., Kawasaki, Y., Matsuura, K., Ueda, H., Tamura, Y., Watanabe, M., Inage, Y., Yakita, Y., Wakabayashi, Y., & Matsumiya, G. (2020). Use of a smart watch for early detection of paroxysmal atrial fibrillation: Validation study. *JMIR Cardio, 4*(1), e14857. https://doi.org/10.2196/14857

Ive, J. (2022). Leveraging the potential of synthetic text for AI in mental healthcare. *Frontiers in Digital Health, 4*, 1010202. https://doi.org/10.3389/fdgth.2022.1010202

Ji, Z., Lee, N., Frieske, R., Yu, T., Su, D., Xu, Y., Ishii, E., Bang, Y., Madotto, A., & Fung, P. (2022). Survey of hallucination in natural language generation. *ACM Computing Surveys*, 3571730. https://doi.org/10.1145/3571730

Kelly, B. S., Judge, C., Bollard, S. M., Clifford, S. M., Healy, G. M., Aziz, A., Mathur, P., Islam, S., Yeom, K. W., Lawlor, A., & Killeen, R. P. (2022). Radiology artificial intelligence: A systematic review and evaluation of methods (RAISE). *European Radiology, 32*(11), 7998–8007. https://doi.org/10.1007/s00330-022-08784-6

Krause, J., Gulshan, V., Rahimy, E., Karth, P., Widner, K., Corrado, G. S., Peng, L., & Webster, D. R. (2018). Grader variability and the importance of reference standards for evaluating machine learning models for diabetic retinopathy. *Ophthalmology, 125*(8), 1264–1272. https://doi.org/10.1016/j.ophtha.2018.01.034

Kundeti, S. R., Vijayananda, J., Mujjiga, S., & Kalyan, M. (2016). Clinical named entity recognition: Challenges and opportunities. *2016 IEEE International Conference on Big Data (Big Data)*, 1937–1945. https://doi.org/10.1109/BigData.2016.7840814

Lee, D. Y., Kim, C., Lee, S., Son, S. J., Cho, S.-M., Cho, Y. H., Lim, J., & Park, R. W. (2022). Psychosis relapse prediction leveraging electronic health records data and natural language processing enrichment methods. *Frontiers in Psychiatry, 13*, 844442. https://doi.org/10.3389/fpsyt.2022.844442

Lee, J. M., & Hauskrecht, M. (2021). Modeling multivariate clinical event time-series with recurrent temporal mechanisms. *Artificial Intelligence in Medicine, 112*, 102021. https://doi.org/10.1016/j.artmed.2021.102021

McKay, C. (2020). Predicting risk in criminal procedure: Actuarial tools, algorithms, AI and judicial decision-making. *Current Issues in Criminal Justice, 32*(1), 22–39. https://doi.org/10.1080/10345329.2019.1658694

Mikolov, T., Chen, K., Corrado, G., & Dean, J. (2013). *Efficient estimation of word representations in vector space.* https://doi.org/10.48550/ARXIV.1301.3781

Muehlematter, U. J., Daniore, P., & Vokinger, K. N. (2021). Approval of artificial intelligence and machine learning-based medical devices in the USA and Europe (2015–20): A comparative analysis. *The Lancet Digital Health*, 3(3), e195–e203. https://doi.org/10.1016/S2589-7500(20)30292-2

Norori, N., Hu, Q., Aellen, F. M., Faraci, F. D., & Tzovara, A. (2021). Addressing bias in big data and AI for health care: A call for open science. *Patterns*, 2(10), 100347. https://doi.org/10.1016/j.patter.2021.100347

Panch, T., Mattie, H., & Celi, L. A. (2019). The "inconvenient truth" about AI in healthcare. *NPJ Digital Medicine*, 2(1), 77. https://doi.org/10.1038/s41746-019-0155-4

Qader, W. A., Ameen, M. M., & Ahmed, B. I. (2019). An overview of bag of words; importance, implementation, applications, and challenges. *2019 International Engineering Conference (IEC)*, 200–204. https://doi.org/10.1109/IEC47844.2019.8950616

Qin, Y., Kernan, K. F., Fan, Z., Park, H.-J., Kim, S., Canna, S. W., Kellum, J. A., Berg, R. A., Wessel, D., Pollack, M. M., Meert, K., Hall, M., Newth, C., Lin, J. C., Doctor, A., Shanley, T., Cornell, T., Harrison, R. E., Zuppa, A. F., … Carcillo, J. A. (2022). Machine learning derivation of four computable 24-h pediatric sepsis phenotypes to facilitate enrollment in early personalized anti-inflammatory clinical trials. *Critical Care*, 26(1), 128. https://doi.org/10.1186/s13054-022-03977-3

Rajpurkar, P., Chen, E., Banerjee, O., & Topol, E. J. (2022). AI in health and medicine. *Nature Medicine*, 28(1), 31–38. https://doi.org/10.1038/s41591-021-01614-0

Rea, F., Corrao, G., Ludergnani, M., Cajazzo, L., & Merlino, L. (2019). A new population-based risk stratification tool was developed and validated for predicting mortality, hospital admissions, and health care costs. *Journal of Clinical Epidemiology*, 116, 62–71. https://doi.org/10.1016/j.jclinepi.2019.08.009

Reddy, S. (2022). Explainability and artificial intelligence in medicine. *The Lancet Digital Health*, 4(4), e214–e215. https://doi.org/10.1016/S2589-7500(22)00029-2

Romero-Brufau, S., Whitford, D., Johnson, M. G., Hickman, J., Morlan, B. W., Therneau, T., Naessens, J., & Huddleston, J. M. (2021). Using machine learning to improve the accuracy of patient deterioration predictions: Mayo Clinic Early Warning Score (MC-EWS). *Journal of the American Medical Informatics Association*, 28(6), 1207–1215. https://doi.org/10.1093/jamia/ocaa347

Russakovsky, O., Deng, J., Su, H., Krause, J., Satheesh, S., Ma, S., Huang, Z., Karpathy, A., Khosla, A., Bernstein, M., Berg, A. C., & Fei-Fei, L. (2015). ImageNet large scale visual recognition challenge. *International Journal of Computer Vision*, 115(3), 211–252. https://doi.org/10.1007/s11263-015-0816-y

Seah, J. C. Y., Tang, C. H. M., Buchlak, Q. D., Holt, X. G., Wardman, J. B., Aimoldin, A., Esmaili, N., Ahmad, H., Pham, H., Lambert, J. F., Hachey, B., Hogg, S. J. F., Johnston, B. P., Bennett, C., Oakden-Rayner, L., Brotchie, P., & Jones, C. M. (2021). Effect of a comprehensive deep-learning model on the accuracy of chest x-ray interpretation by radiologists: A retrospective, multireader multicase study. *The Lancet Digital Health*, 3(8), e496–e506. https://doi.org/10.1016/S2589-7500(21)00106-0

Searle, T., Ibrahim, Z., Teo, J., & Dobson, R. (2022). *Summarisation of electronic health records with clinical concept guidance.* https://doi.org/10.48550/ARXIV.2211.07126

Shwartz-Ziv, R., & Armon, A. (2021). *Tabular data: Deep learning is not all you need.* https://doi.org/10.48550/ARXIV.2106.03253

Sipari, D., Chaparro-Rico, B. D. M., & Cafolla, D. (2022). SANE (Easy Gait Analysis System): Towards an AI-assisted automatic gait-analysis. *International Journal of Environmental Research and Public Health*, 19(16), 10032. https://doi.org/10.3390/ijerph191610032

Teo, J. T. H., Dinu, V., Bernal, W., Davidson, P., Oliynyk, V., Breen, C., Barker, R. D., & Dobson, R. J. B. (2021). Real-time clinician text feeds from electronic health records. *NPJ Digital Medicine*, *4*(1), 35. https://doi.org/10.1038/s41746-021-00406-7

The INFORM-lab, Palmer, E., Klapaukh, R., Harris, S., & Singer, M. (2019). Intelligently learning from data. *Critical Care*, *23*(1). https://doi.org/10.1186/s13054-019-2424-7

Tilmes, N. (2022). Disability, fairness, and algorithmic bias in AI recruitment. *Ethics and Information Technology*, *24*(2), 21. https://doi.org/10.1007/s10676-022-09633-2

Topol, E. J. (2019). High-performance medicine: The convergence of human and artificial intelligence. *Nature Medicine*, *25*(1), 44–56. https://doi.org/10.1038/s41591-018-0300-7

Tsui, F. R., Shi, L., Ruiz, V., Ryan, N. D., Biernesser, C., Iyengar, S., Walsh, C. G., & Brent, D. A. (2021). Natural language processing and machine learning of electronic health records for prediction of first-time suicide attempts. *JAMIA Open*, *4*(1), ooab011. https://doi.org/10.1093/jamiaopen/ooab011

Voelker, R. (2020). Cardiac ultrasound uses artificial intelligence to produce images. *JAMA*, *323*(11), 1034. https://doi.org/10.1001/jama.2020.2547

Whang, S. E., Roh, Y., Song, H., & Lee, J.-G. (2021). *Data collection and quality challenges in deep learning: A data-centric AI perspective*. https://doi.org/10.48550/ARXIV.2112.06409

Whebell, S., & Zhang, J. (2022). Bringing biological ARDS phenotypes to the bedside with machine-learning-based classifiers. *The Lancet Respiratory Medicine*, *10*(4), 319–320. https://doi.org/10.1016/S2213-2600(21)00492-6

Wong, A., Otles, E., Donnelly, J. P., Krumm, A., McCullough, J., DeTroyer-Cooley, O., Pestrue, J., Phillips, M., Konye, J., Penoza, C., Ghous, M., & Singh, K. (2021). External validation of a widely implemented proprietary sepsis prediction model in hospitalized patients. *JAMA Internal Medicine*, *181*(8), 1065. https://doi.org/10.1001/jamainternmed.2021.2626

Wu, S., Roberts, K., Datta, S., Du, J., Ji, Z., Si, Y., Soni, S., Wang, Q., Wei, Q., Xiang, Y., Zhao, B., & Xu, H. (2020). Deep learning in clinical natural language processing: A methodical review. *Journal of the American Medical Informatics Association*, *27*(3), 457–470. https://doi.org/10.1093/jamia/ocz200

Yamashita, R., Nishio, M., Do, R. K. G., & Togashi, K. (2018). Convolutional neural networks: An overview and application in radiology. *Insights into Imaging*, *9*(4), 611–629. https://doi.org/10.1007/s13244-018-0639-9

Yang, X., Bian, J., Hogan, W. R., & Wu, Y. (2020). Clinical concept extraction using transformers. *Journal of the American Medical Informatics Association*, *27*(12), 1935–1942. https://doi.org/10.1093/jamia/ocaa189

Yu, S. C., Shivakumar, N., Betthauser, K., Gupta, A., Lai, A. M., Kollef, M. H., Payne, P. R. O., & Michelson, A. P. (2021). Comparison of early warning scores for sepsis early identification and prediction in the general ward setting. *JAMIA Open*, *4*(3), ooab062. https://doi.org/10.1093/jamiaopen/ooab062

Zhang, J., Budhdeo, S., William, W., Cerrato, P., Shuaib, H., Sood, H., Ashrafian, H., Halamka, J., & Teo, J. T. (2022). Moving towards vertically integrated artificial intelligence development. *NPJ Digital Medicine*, *5*(1), 143. https://doi.org/10.1038/s41746-022-00690-x

Zhang, J., Mattie, H., Shuaib, H., Hensman, T., Teo, J. T., & Celi, L. A. (2022). Addressing the "elephant in the room" of AI clinical decision support through organisation-level regulation. *PLOS Digital Health*, *1*(9), e0000111. https://doi.org/10.1371/journal.pdig.0000111

Zhang, J., Symons, J., Agapow, P., Teo, J. T., Paxton, C. A., Abdi, J., Mattie, H., Davie, C., Torres, A. Z., Folarin, A., Sood, H., Celi, L. A., Halamka, J., Eapen, S., & Budhdeo, S. (2022). Best practices in the real-world data life cycle. *PLOS Digital Health*, *1*(1), e0000003. https://doi.org/10.1371/journal.pdig.0000003

Zhang, J., Whebell, S., Gallifant, J., Budhdeo, S., Mattie, H., Lertvittayakumjorn, P., del Pilar Arias Lopez, M., Tiangco, B. J., Gichoya, J. W., Ashrafian, H., Celi, L. A., & Teo, J. T. (2022).

An interactive dashboard to track themes, development maturity, and global equity in clinical artificial intelligence research. *The Lancet Digital Health*, 4(4), e212–e213. https://doi.org/10.1016/S2589-7500(22)00032-2

Zhang, J., Whebell, S. F., Sanderson, B., Retter, A., Daly, K., Paul, R., Barrett, N., Agarwal, S., Lams, B. E., Meadows, C., Terblanche, M., & Camporota, L. (2021). Phenotypes of severe COVID-19 ARDS receiving extracorporeal membrane oxygenation. *British Journal of Anaesthesia*, 126(3), e130–e132. https://doi.org/10.1016/j.bja.2020.12.023

3

The Need for AI in Healthcare

Vince Madai

Charité Universitätsmedizin, Berlin, Germany

LEARNING OBJECTIVES

- Understand the current challenges for healthcare systems
- Describe the concept of healthcare sustainability
- Describe the challenges to healthcare sustainability
- Describe how digital technologies, in particular AI, can increase healthcare system sustainability
- Evaluate why AI is specifically needed in the areas of administration, finance, operations, and clinical care

---

Introduction

Artificial Intelligence (AI) is finding increasing application in a variety of industries. One example is the use of large language models such as GPT-3, which can be used for natural language processing tasks such as language translation, text summarisation and question answering. One prominent example is the recently introduced ChatGPT service, an advanced AI chatbot. Other examples of the use of AI in industry include self-driving cars that use AI to navigate and make decisions in traffic (Parekh et al., 2022), or financial services where AI is used to detect and prevent fraud (Sengupta et al., 2018).

Considering this widespread use, the use of AI in healthcare seems like a logical next step. However, in an ethically sensitive area like healthcare, we should be careful in using a new technology just because it is fashionable or hyped. We need to consider the opportunity costs in allocating limited funds to a new technology: Why was the money spent on this new technology and not on other technologies or more standard interventions and solutions? Therefore, we must first answer important questions before applying AI in healthcare: Do we need AI in healthcare? And if so, why?

The area where there would be significant impact of AI tools in healthcare, will be our healthcare systems. This is an important aspect since it is tempting to dive headlong into the discussion of a singular technology whilst losing the big picture. The big picture *are* our healthcare systems that comprise the totality of organizations, people, and actions

DOI: 10.1201/9781003262152-3

that promote, restore, or maintain health (World Health Organization = Organisation mondiale de la Santé, 2007). To reach this goal, healthcare systems engage in activities that include the direct provision of health services to people and populations, ranging from prevention to treatment or rehabilitation. They also include the necessary activities that aim at providing the resources for the functioning of healthcare systems, e.g, financial resources. Globally, we can observe very differently organised types of healthcare systems. However, the overarching goal of all healthcare systems is to maintain and improve the health of citizens in the most effective and efficient way (World Health Organization, 2007).

We can observe, however, that healthcare systems around the world are struggling to achieve this goal. If we continue the current path, we will soon be unable to provide the required level of care, not only in low- or middle-income countries, but also in high-income countries. As a result, we can expect a significant impact on the accessibility to and the quality of healthcare services, and novel treatments will increasingly only be available to wealthy patients. As a result, one of the most pressing healthcare policy challenges is to at least maintain the level of care in our present-day healthcare systems. **Maintaining the status quo of a system is called sustainability** and considering healthcare we can state that the sustainability of our healthcare systems is at great risk.

Thus, we urgently need to find approaches to increase the sustainability of healthcare systems. In this context, we can find the main argument for the need to AI in healthcare. In general, new digital technologies have the potential to increase the effectiveness and/or efficiency of services in all areas of healthcare. AI is one of the most promising approaches of this group of novel digital technologies, and why we need more AI in our healthcare systems is the main subject of this chapter.

This chapter is structured as follows. It first introduces the concept of healthcare system sustainability in more detail. Then it presents the main threats to healthcare system sustainability and outlines how AI can increase sustainability. Finally, the chapter concludes by presenting the concrete needs for promising AI applications in the main healthcare areas of administration, finance, operations, and clinical care.

Healthcare System Sustainability

When we refer to "Healthcare System Sustainability", we mainly mean the ability of a healthcare system to maintain the activities and services that are required to provide the adequate level of care for all citizens. Based on the summary of the literature provided by Lennox et al. (Lennox et al., 2018), sustainability should not, however, be seen as a static metric that is only focused on measuring whether or not the level of services is still adequate. Rather, the ability to adapt, react, and to improve when facing challenges has also been recognized as being an integral part of sustainability. Thus, instead of a static metric, sustainability should be seen as a process with continuous development. Based on these considerations, Lennox et al also provide a definition of sustainability: "*The general continuation and maintenance of a desirable feature of an initiative and its associated outcomes as well as the process taken to adapt and develop in response to emerging needs of the system*".

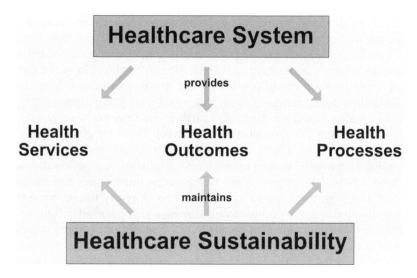

FIGURE 3.1
Healthcare system and sustainability.

(Source: Author.)

To make this definition more accessible, especially for our healthcare needs, we can rephrase the above-introduced definition as follows: *"Healthcare sustainability is the general continuation and maintenance of a desired level of health services and health outcomes as well as the processes taken to adapt and develop in response to emerging needs and threats of health care systems."* As we can see, the three main factors of healthcare sustainability are *health services*, *health outcomes*, and *processes* (see Figure 3.1): Desired levels of health services can be, for example, the availability of General Practitioners and/or medical specialists per capita, and their availability in rural areas. Health outcomes can be morbidity and mortality rates during childbirth or for diseases such as cancer, stroke, or heart attack. Processes may involve (long-term) administrative processes and other strategies to improve the efficiency of healthcare systems. We will see in the next section that there are major threats to healthcare system sustainability that simultaneously affect all three: health services, health outcomes, and processes.

Health systems provide health services through health processes that lead to specific health outcomes. Health system sustainability aims to maintain the desired level for all three aspects.

Threats to Healthcare System Sustainability

The primary threat to healthcare sustainability are rapidly ageing populations. With increasing age, the incidence of diseases increases, leading to a rising demand for healthcare services. Globally, the population of citizens aged 65 and above is projected to increase from 10% in 2022 to 16% in 2050 (*World Population Prospects 2022: Summary of Results*, n.d.). In absolute terms, this is an increase from 800 million to 1.5 billion people given the overall increase in global population (*World Population Prospects 2022: Summary of Results*, n.d.). Such ageing populations are primarily associated with high-income countries, where the effects of ageing are already visible. However, the most rapidly ageing populations are found outside of high-income countries. Measures such as improved sanitation, better access to clean water and food, campaigns aimed at disease prevention, vaccinations, and a reduction of birth-related deaths have greatly increased the odds to lead a longer life (Amalberti et al., 2016). Thus, by 2050, two-thirds of the world´s population above 60 will be found in low- and middle-income countries (*Ageing and Health*, n.d.). This means that in high-income countries, increasing the sustainability of healthcare systems is, in part, a reactive process, but in low- and middle-income countries there is a high need for prospective action. Already today, more than three-quarters of deaths due to non-communicable diseases are observed in low- and middle-income countries (*Noncommunicable Diseases*, n.d.). Consequently, there is a major need to rapidly tackle the effects of ageing in high-income countries and prepare low- and middle-income countries for the wave of elderly patients with their complex health needs. How exactly, however, does ageing negatively affect sustainability? We have previously established that the relevant factors for sustainability are health services, health outcomes, and health processes. So, we can use these three categories to answer this question.

First, ageing increases the demand for healthcare services. It increases the risk for acute and chronic diseases with a high disease and economic burden such as cardio- and cerebrovascular diseases or cancer: In the western world, the lifetime risk for stroke, for example, has reached almost 25% for some countries ("Global, Regional, and Country-Specific Lifetime Risks of Stroke, 1990 and 2016," 2018; Phan et al., 2020), and the lifetime risk for some cancer types has risen to around 40% (*Lifetime Risk of Developing or Dying From Cancer* https://www.Cancer.Org/Cancer/Cancer-Basics/Lifetime-Probability-of-Developing-or-Dying-from-Cancer.Html, 2020). These diseases are complex and require interdisciplinary and interconnected care involving multiple disciplines and institutions. The delivery of healthcare services under these conditions is further complicated as ageing decreases the ability to access healthcare services via impairments of sensory and cognitive functions. These include hearing loss, cataracts, osteoarthritis, depression, and dementia, which, in turn, lead to complex geriatric syndromes that are accompanied by frailty, urinary incontinence, falls, deliriums and pressure ulcers (*Ageing and Health*, n.d.). Often, several major and minor health conditions are present in a single elderly patient; this is what is known as co-morbidity. The provision of adequate health services for ageing patients is further aggravated by the fact that such populations also lead to shortage of healthcare staff. More and extended healthcare needs would require an increase of healthcare staff to meet the demand. Ageing populations limit the available workforce. For OECD countries, researchers forecast a shortage of 400,000 doctors and 2.5 million nurses as early as the year 2030 (Scheffler & Arnold, 2019). This also poses major challenges for the training of new doctors: There will be a rising demand for generalist knowledge to deal with the multiple co-morbidities of elderly patients, and to be able to treat patients holistically (Rimmer, 2017). On the other hand, however, there is a projected major shortage of specialists, especially in highly sensitive areas such as hospice and palliative medicine which are required for the ageing population (Lupu et al., 2018). These contradictory demands cannot be met with a decreasing workforce.

A further challenge for health services provision is the fact that the rising costs resulting from the increasing demand for service and innovative progress cannot be met by the available budgets. In all OECD countries, for example, health spending has exceeded economic growth for decades (OECD, 2015). This leads to a decrease of available services - when an increase is warranted - with catastrophic consequences, especially for vulnerable sub-populations such as the elderly.

Ageing is also a detriment to health outcomes. During the ageing process of the human body, various physiological changes occur that can have a detrimental effect on health outcomes. The ageing process is associated with a decrease in immune function, which leads to an increased susceptibility to infections and the development of cancer. In addition, age increases the risk of chronic diseases such as cardiovascular disease, diabetes mellitus, and stroke. Bone density decreases with advancing age, leading to increased susceptibility to osteoporotic fractures. In addition, muscle mass and function decrease, increasing the risk of falls and related injuries. Cognitive decline and memory loss are also associated with ageing, as mentioned previously. Further, less and less doctors need to deal with increasing numbers of patients with complex health needs. The result is a strained and stressed workforce that works constantly at its limits. Under such conditions, doctors experience detriments to their own health, mainly burnouts (Lemaire & Wallace, 2017). This condition has become so prevalent that it has been called a public health crisis (Noseworthy et al., n.d.). Unsurprisingly, more medical errors occur in such an environment (West et al., 2009). This is also a major threat to the maintenance of the workforce. In the UK NHS, for example, a growing number of doctors are considering to leave the NHS, or medicine altogether, citing excessive workloads and financial reasons (Lambert et al., 2018).

Lastly, ageing also affects health processes and this fact is inextricably tied to the question of efficiency in our healthcare systems. The challenges to health services and outcomes due to ageing put additional pressure on healthcare processes to be efficient. This is particularly important y when we consider the required and interconnected care necessary for people with co-morbidities, where patients need to regularly see healthcare specialists from multiple domains in a systematic fashion. In reality, we already see major inefficiencies in the currently applied models of healthcare. The OECD reports that 30% of total health expenditure in its member countries is due to waste (OECD, 2017). Doctors are fighting bureaucracy whose intention it is to keep costs within budgets, while doctors try to navigate the bureaucracy to provide the best possible care for patients (Lorkowski et al., 2021). Waste in this situation can be defined as either services that are harmful or do not provide benefits or costs that could be avoided by replacing a service with another that is cheaper but as effective (OECD, 2017). A major contributing factor to waste are poorly organized and managed healthcare systems (OECD, 2017). The problem, however, is not only the status quo but the outlook: The current centralized and rather inflexible care models will struggle to keep up with the novel challenges posed by an ageing population (Braithwaite et al., 2018). But we also need to be careful when trying to battle waste: Excessive documentation, information overload, and over-reliance on bureaucratic metrics, called the "McDonaldization of medicine", can lead to the opposite effects (Dorsey & Ritzer, 2016).

In summary, current healthcare systems applying inefficient and outdated models of care will not be able to keep up with the challenges posed by population increase and population ageing. Health services will provide less and less benefits, health outcomes will deteriorate, and health services will become increasingly inefficient. This is a global phenomenon that will become prevalent in high-income countries earlier, but will also eventually hit low- and middle-income countries with full force. Thus, new models of care are urgently needed to tackle these challenges.

AI to Increase Healthcare System Sustainability

The previously mentioned challenges have been met with ideas to tackle them. Mainly, in the form of health policy suggestion on how to increase healthcare system sustainability. In general, we can find the majority of healthcare strategy and policy recommendations not in peer-reviewed academic literature but in policy documents by international governance organizations and think tanks (Braithwaite et al., 2019). Overall, these recommendations agree that digital innovation will increase the quality of health services, will lead to better health outcomes, and will increase health process efficiency. For example, the European Union-supported European Institute of Innovation and Technology (EIT) Health Thinktank identified digitalization, data and technology innovation as a key area to build sustainable healthcare systems in Europe (EITH ThinkTank, 2022). The Partnership for Health Sustainability and Resilience (PHSSR) highlighted that technological innovations may offer significant benefits to foster healthcare sustainability, through transformative positive impacts and the utilisation of digital health services (WEF, n.d.).

In this context, AI is one of the most promising examples of current digital innovation playing a prominent role in predictions on how digital health will transform health care. For example, in a report by Deloitte it was estimated that the widespread application of AI could save, annually, approximately 400,000 lives, 200 billion euros, and 1.8 billion working hours in the European Union alone (Deloitte, 2020). For the US, it was estimated that within 5 years up to 360 billion dollars could be saved annually, if existing technology was to be rolled out widely (Sahni et al., 2023). The World Innovation Summit for Health (WISH) report calls AI a tool of the 21st century and highlights how the increasing generation of data sets the ground for AI-based transformation of the healthcare systems worldwide (Colclough et al., n.d.). EIT Health and McKinsey, for example, focus specifically how AI will change the structure of the healthcare workforce across the dimensions of shifts in employment structure and changes in the activities of the workforce, for example reducing administrative tasks (*Eit-Health-and-Mckinsey_transforming-Healthcare-with-Ai.Pdf*, n.d.). And finally, the Topol review stressed how AI may transform the UK NHS by streamlining processes, improving diagnostic accuracy and helping staff work more efficiently (*HEE-Topol-Review-2019.pdf*, n.d.). The UK NHS serves also as a case study in this chapter (see case study box).

However, we need to be careful with the uptake of such non-peer-reviewed reports, authored by institutions outside of academia. The application of novel technologies in healthcare is not necessarily a panacea. Non-academic reports are likely to be overly optimistic in their forecasting since their authors are not unbiased, generally having monetary interests considering the implementation of new technologies. Especially with an ageing population in mind, digital innovation, and thus AI solutions, can also increase costs, if not done in a strategically optimal way. As the population ages, demand increases for healthcare services specifically designed for older adults, such as treatments for age-related diseases and technologies that facilitate mobility and daily living. This increased demand may also drive up costs as healthcare providers and manufacturers can charge more for these specialised services and products. In addition, many new technologies and treatments developed with an ageing population in mind may be more expensive than the existing options due to the cost of research and development. This can also increase costs for older adults as they are more likely to use these specialised treatments and technologies. This shows that innovative new technologies must be embedded in an overall digitalization and sustainability strategy, as otherwise unwanted effects may counter potential benefits. Also, the development of AI tools for healthcare should follow clearly outlined best practices for technical and ethical development ensuring the highest level of validation and impact (Higgins & Madai, 2020; McCradden et al., 2022; Zhang et al., 2022b).

Importantly, we also need to translate these high-level needs, the general need for AI in healthcare, to target needs in specific areas. To this end, this chapter will follow the structure of the expert panel of the American Hospital Association that surveyed the AI health care landscape (American Hospital Association, n.d.). They divided the AI landscape into the areas of administration, finance, operations, and clinical delivery (see Figure 3.2). Considering the last point, the chapter will also mention the relevant need for AI in healthcare from the specific perspective of low- and middle-income countries versus high-income countries, as their needs in the distinct areas can differ considerably. For example, in Africa, there is a lack of availability of infrastructure that is readily available in high-income countries. The penetration of mobile phones, however, is expected to reach 100% within the next decades, an emphasis on solutions developed for mobile phone use rather than desktops (Owoyemi et al., 2020).

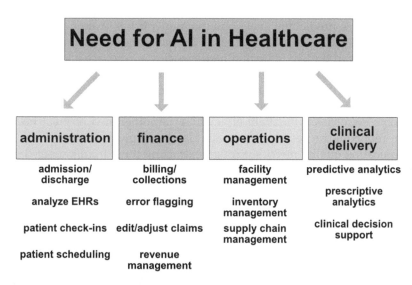

FIGURE 3.2
Need for AI in healthcare. (Adapted from American Hospital Association, n.d.)

The Need for AI in Administration

In general, administrative tasks have a critical role in healthcare processes, and secondary effects on the availability of health services. The idea that administrative tasks need to be improved and that this need can be met by AI is a widespread view (Reddy et al., 2019). When considering such administrative tasks, AI is tailor-made for those specific tasks that share the following six characteristics: they are manual, repetitive, transactional, defined by limited data elements, rely on structured data and generate abundant data (American Hospital Association, n.d.). For example, AI improvements are needed in admission and discharge procedures. In many healthcare systems, admissions and discharges are accompanied with an excessive amount of paperwork (Caldwell, 2023). Natural language processing (NLP)-based tools could be developed that are able to analyze large amount of electronic health record (EHR) information and can organize them for doctors and patients alike (Gilvaz et al., 2019). Such systems can be used to pre-populate an online form with information from the EHR and billing system and can inform all caregivers and departments that the patient is on site to prepare them for the delivery of health services (American Hospital Association, n.d.). A similar area where bureaucratic paperwork could be reduced are discharge documents and instructions that can also be improved with AI. By eliminating standard paper forms and replacing them with customized instructions based on an individual patient's health status and treatment plan, patients could get better personalized information and could access the instructions electronically through an app on their smartphones, making the process more efficient and patient-centered (American Hospital Association, n.d.).

When considering the need of patient-centeredness, patients' check-in procedures can also be improved with AI. By using a self-check-in process when patients arrive for scheduled outpatient visits, an AI system can automatically recognize patients and engage in an AI-driven chat session, which is automatically fed into the EHR (American Hospital Association, n.d.). Another example with a major need is appointment scheduling. An AI system may spot when patients' and providers' appointment availability aligns and could also predict the likelihood that patients fail to attend scheduled hospital visits (Nelson et al., 2019), making it easier for patients and healthcare staff to schedule appointments and thereby reducing inefficiencies in resource allocation (American Hospital Association, n.d.). An example for a complex ward-and-bed allocation system can be found in the work of Mellouli and Stoeck (Mellouli & Stoeck, 2021).

AI-based resource management systems have also been tested successfully in low-and middle-income countries (Munavalli et al., 2021). Another area of great need is quality measure reporting processes, which can also be improved with AI. By capturing and communicating quality metrics through extracting them from patient data, and by knowing which metrics to use for individual health plans and value-based reimbursement models and transmitting them electronically to the appropriate users and payers, AI can help improve the accuracy and efficiency of reporting quality metrics (American Hospital Association, n.d.). Areas with lesser but still relevant needs are, for example, customer service responses that can also benefit from AI technology. By giving patients 24/7 access to the information they need, AI can help to improve patient satisfaction and reduce the workload for customer service staff (American Hospital Association, n.d.). Or hiring and orientation protocols that can also be streamlined with AI. By automating routine and transactional human resources functions, AI can help to speed up the hiring process and reduce the workload for HR staff (American Hospital Association, n.d.). Overall, the use of AI in administration can help to improve the efficiency and accuracy of various administrative tasks, reduce the workload for staff and make all processes more patient-centered (American Hospital Association, n.d.).

The Need for AI in Finance

Financial tasks are usually less in the spotlight, when AI in healthcare applications is discussed. They are, however, a prime example of healthcare processes, where there is a need for efficiency gains to save costs. Given the repetitive nature of finance processes and the already existing automation and digitalization of the data, AI can play a major role to meet this need. A main area where AI can be particularly useful is in billing and collections. By generating accurate and timely bills for patients, healthcare organizations can reduce costs and increase receivables (American Hospital Association, n.d.). Additionally, AI can also be used to identify and flag any errors or inconsistencies in the billing process, reducing the likelihood of denied claims and payment delays. Another area where there is a need for AI is in claims management. There is a need for AI systems that can edit and adjust claims to produce a clean claim, reducing payment delays and denials. This can be achieved by analyzing claims data and identifying patterns that indicate errors or inconsistencies, such as missing information or incorrect codes (American Hospital Association, n.d.). Here, there are also solutions in use that are tailored to the specific needs of low- and middle-income countries (Eke et al., 2023). Moreover, organizations could replace manual processes with AI-powered automated tools to address fraud, waste and abuse (FWA) (Sahni et al., 2023). Lastly, revenue cycle management is another area where AI can be applied to improve financial healthcare. By using AI to see in real time what's coming in from each patient by type of health plan, healthcare organizations can improve the accuracy of financial projections and speed up monthly closes (American Hospital Association, n.d.). In conclusion, AI has the potential to meet the needs in financial healthcare operations by streamlining financial processes to increase efficiency.

The Need for AI in Healthcare Operations

In modern healthcare, the need for efficient and effective operations is crucial. This is another area that mainly affects healthcare processes but can also indirectly affect access to healthcare services, and even health outcomes. One of the major areas where AI in healthcare operations is needed is facilities management. Predictive maintenance is a powerful tool that can help reduce operational costs by predicting when equipment needs to be serviced or replaced to make better-informed decisions about when to replace equipment (American Hospital Association, n.d.). Materials and inventory management is another area where there is a need for AI and it can have a significant impact. By tracking, analyzing, and reporting all goods, medical supplies, equipment, devices, and technology across an enterprise, healthcare providers can optimize their use and reduce losses (American Hospital Association, n.d.). Also, AI-based systems can be used to monitor energy consumption and predict failures in medical devices, allowing healthcare providers to take proactive measures to prevent disruptions (American Hospital Association, n.d.). Finally, supply chain management is another area where AI is needed. By capturing true case costs and alerting staff when expected supplies aren't on the consumption report, healthcare providers can improve cost-variance analysis and procedure and inventory-demand intelligence. AI-based systems can also present the relationship between supply variances and patient outcomes, allowing healthcare providers to identify areas where they can improve patient outcomes while reducing costs (American Hospital Association, n.d.). In conclusion, AI may meet the needs of various operational aspects by reducing costs and by improving efficiency. As a result access to healthcare services can be optimized, and even health outcomes may be improved by making sure that facilities operate efficiently, and all required medical materials and goods are readily available. Specifically, in low- and middle-income countries there may be further needs, such as AI-powered solutions to battle the sale of counterfeit medicine through AI-based real-time verification of pharmaceuticals (Eke et al., 2023). Reuter-Opperman and Kühl provide an overview of further examples of AI in healthcare operations (Reuter-Oppermann & Kühl, 2021).

The Need for AI in Clinical Delivery

The last major area with a need for AI solutions is the area of clinical delivery, which principally affects health outcomes but also affects the efficient working of health services. The need for AI in healthcare can be subdivided into the need for predictive and so-called prescriptive analytics. Predictive analytics are the AI methods that take historic data as an input and provide information about future trends, behaviour and activity (Deshpande et al., 2019). Prescriptive analytics, on the other hand, aims at solving a dilemma: For certain use cases it might not be sufficient to know what will likely happen in the future but we also want information on the right course of action based on the prediction when several courses of action are available (Deshpande et al., 2019). Examples for the need for predictive use cases would be to predict the prevalence of a disease or the mortality rates of certain cancer types (Lopes et al., 2020). Or the need for triaging cases, identifying vulnerable patients in need of navigation services, and combinations of AI and wearable technologies for remote monitoring. These technologies can help identify patients at risk, provide personalized health management and provide clinical insights from multiple sources to improve patient outcomes. Considering prescriptive analytics in healthcare, there is a need for tools that provide clinical decision support in the form of information which medical intervention to favor in certain predictive scenarios. For example, these tools might help clinicians diagnose diseases and recommend customized treatment plans based on the latest evidence-based medical guidelines and the patient's unique characteristics, such as biomarkers and genes (American Hospital Association, n.d.). Specifically, these solutions can be applied in the areas of automated image interpretation, genomic diagnostics, interventional and rehabilitative robotics, precision/personalized medicine, and telemedicine for remote patient monitoring (American Hospital Association, n.d.). Importantly, in low- and middle-income countries increasingly local companies have begun to develop solutions specifically tailored to the needs of their populations, for example for eye disease screening or skin disease diagnosis and treatment recommendation for darker skin types (Eke et al., 2023).

CASE STUDY THE UK NATIONAL HEALTH SYSTEM (NHS)

- The **National Health Service (NHS)** of the United Kingdom (UK) is a publicly funded healthcare system that provides comprehensive healthcare for all UK citizens. However, the NHS is currently facing **major challenges** in the face of an **ageing population**. Demographic change is putting a strain on the NHS, as older people tend to have **more chronic diseases and are more likely to need medical care**.
- At the same time, the **shortage of medical staff** is an additional challenge for the NHS. This is due to an **ageing workforce**, with many experienced doctors and nurses approaching retirement age. There is also a growing **shortage of GPs**, making it increasingly difficult for patients to access primary care services. In addition to these challenges, the NHS is also struggling with **financial problems**. In recent years, the NHS has faced budgetary constraints, leading to cuts in services and staff. This has led to longer waiting times for patients and limited access to certain treatments.
- In the face of these challenges, digital technology, particularly **Artificial Intelligence (AI)**, has the potential to help the NHS become more sustainable. To this end, the NHS has launched the **NHS AI Lab**, a programme that promotes **collaboration and co-development** to lower the barriers to the **development and deployment of AI systems** in the NHS. The Lab has a conceptual **roadmap**, dedicated **funding programmes** for development and evaluation, and has as of 2023 already **delivered five AI tools** to improve the efficiency and accuracy of health processes, services and clinical care.
- In summary, the UK NHS, like all other health systems, faces major challenges related to the ageing population. With a dedicated programme and roadmap for AI in healthcare, the NHS is seeking to harness the benefits of AI to make the NHS more sustainable by improving the efficiency of healthcare services and reducing costs.

Conclusion

Ageing populations pose an unsurmountable challenge to the sustainability of our healthcare systems if we try to tackle this problem using current approaches. AI technology has immense potential to increase and guarantee the sustainability of healthcare systems by improving efficacy and efficiency. The chapter identified specific needs for AI in healthcare can be identified for four main areas of healthcare, namely administration, finance, operations, and clinical care, as well as for low- and middle-income countries. The application of AI in healthcare, however, is not a panacea. It should be strategically embedded in a comprehensive digitization and sustainability strategy, and AI tools should follow clearly outlined best practices for technical and ethical development.

SUMMARY

- Healthcare systems need to maintain desired levels of health processes, services and outcomes, i.e. they need to be sustainable.
- The rapidly ageing population and its secondary effects such as increased costs and labor shortage are a major threat to healthcare system sustainability.
- AI can help make healthcare systems sustainable by increasing the efficiency of health processes, by making healthcare services more effective and efficient, and by improving health outcomes.
- AI is needed in the four main areas of administration, finance, operations, and clinical care.
- The application of AI in healthcare should be strategically embedded in a comprehensive digitization and sustainability strategy, and AI tools should follow clearly outlined best practices for technical and ethical development.

REVIEW QUESTIONS

- How does ageing affect our healthcare systems? Name at least three important aspects.
- Why is the sustainability of healthcare important? What would happen if our healthcare systems were no longer sustainable?
- How can we define sustainability in healthcare? Why is it difficult to define?
- How can digital health and especially Artificial Intelligence support the sustainability of healthcare systems?
- Define at least three specific areas with examples where there is a need for AI solutions in healthcare

Bibliography

Acosta, J. N., Falcone, G. J., Rajpurkar, P., & Topol, E. J. (2022). Multimodal biomedical AI. *Nature Medicine, 28*(9), 1773–1784. https://doi.org/10.1038/s41591-022-01981-2

Ageing and health. (n.d.). Retrieved November 27, 2022, from https://www.who.int/news-room/fact-sheets/detail/ageing-and-health

Amalberti, R., Nicklin, W., & Braithwaite, J. (2016). Preparing national health systems to cope with the impending tsunami of ageing and its associated complexities: Towards more sustainable health care. *International Journal for Quality in Health Care, 28*(3), 412–414. https://doi.org/10.1093/intqhc/mzw021

American Hospital Association. (n.d.). *Surveying the AI Health Care Landscape.* Retrieved October 31, 2022, from https://www.aha.org/system/files/media/file/2019/10/Market_Insights_AI-Landscape.pdf

Andrew, Ng. (2021, June). *MLOps: From model-centric to data-centric AI.* https://www.deeplearning.ai/wp-content/uploads/2021/06/MLOps-From-Model-centric-to-Data-centric-AI.pdf

Beede, E., Baylor, E., Hersch, F., Iurchenko, A., Wilcox, L., Ruamviboonsuk, P., & Vardoulakis, L. M. (2020). A human-centered evaluation of a deep learning system deployed in clinics for the detection of diabetic retinopathy. *Proceedings of the 2020 CHI Conference on Human Factors in Computing Systems*, 1–12. https://doi.org/10.1145/3313831.3376718

Benson, T., & Grieve, G. (2016). *Principles of health interoperability: SNOMED CT, HL7 and FHIR*. Springer International Publishing. https://doi.org/10.1007/978-3-319-30370-3

Bhatia, P., Celikkaya, B., Khalilia, M., & Senthivel, S. (2019). Comprehend medical: A named entity recognition and relationship extraction web service. *2019 18th IEEE International Conference On Machine Learning And Applications (ICMLA)*, 1844–1851. https://doi.org/10.1109/ICMLA.2019.00297

Braithwaite, J., Mannion, R., Matsuyama, Y., Shekelle, P. G., Whittaker, S., Al-Adawi, S., Ludlow, K., James, W., Ting, H. P., Herkes, J., McPherson, E., Churruca, K., Lamprell, G., Ellis, L. A., Boyling, C., Warwick, M., Pomare, C., Nicklin, W., & Hughes, C. F. (2018). The future of health systems to 2030: A roadmap for global progress and sustainability. *International Journal for Quality in Health Care*, 30(10), 823–831. https://doi.org/10.1093/intqhc/mzy242

Braithwaite, J., Zurynski, Y., Ludlow, K., Holt, J., Augustsson, H., & Campbell, M. (2019). Towards sustainable healthcare system performance in the 21st century in high-income countries: A protocol for a systematic review of the grey literature. *BMJ Open*, 9(1), e025892. https://doi.org/10.1136/bmjopen-2018-025892

Bzdok, D., Altman, N., & Krzywinski, M. (2018). Statistics versus machine learning. *Nature Methods*, 15(4), 233–234. https://doi.org/10.1038/nmeth.4642

Caldwell, G. (2023, January 28). *The NHS is drowning in paperwork*. The Spectator. https://www.spectator.co.uk/article/the-nhs-is-drowning-in-paperwork/

Cho, S.-Y., Kim, S.-H., Kang, S.-H., Lee, K. J., Choi, D., Kang, S., Park, S. J., Kim, T., Yoon, C.-H., Youn, T.-J., & Chae, I.-H. (2021). Pre-existing and machine learning-based models for cardiovascular risk prediction. *Scientific Reports*, 11(1), 8886. https://doi.org/10.1038/s41598-021-88257-w

Colclough, G., Dorling, G., Riahi, F., Ghafur, S., & Sheikh, A. (n.d.). *Harnessing Data Science and AI in Healthcare - From Policy to Practice*.

Conway, M., Hu, M., & Chapman, W. W. (2019). Recent advances in using natural language processing to address public health research questions using social media and consumer generated data. *Yearbook of Medical Informatics*, 28(01), 208–217. https://doi.org/10.1055/s-0039-1677918

Côté, M. J., & Smith, M. A. (2018). Forecasting the demand for radiology services. *Health Systems*, 7(2), 79–88. https://doi.org/10.1080/20476965.2017.1390056

Cui, M., & Zhang, D. Y. (2021). Artificial intelligence and computational pathology. *Laboratory Investigation*, 101(4), 412–422. https://doi.org/10.1038/s41374-020-00514-0

Deloitte. (2020). *The socio-economic impact of AI in healthcare*. https://www.medtecheurope.org/wp-content/uploads/2020/10/mte-ai_impact-in-healthcare_oct2020_report.pdf

Deshpande, P. S., Sharma, S. C., & Peddoju, S. K. (2019). Predictive and prescriptive analytics in big-data era. In P. S. Deshpande, S. C. Sharma, & S. K. Peddoju (Eds.), *Security and data storage aspect in cloud computing* (pp. 71–81). Springer. https://doi.org/10.1007/978-981-13-6089-3_5

Dismuke, C. (2020). Progress in examining cost-effectiveness of AI in diabetic retinopathy screening. *The Lancet Digital Health*, 2(5), e212–e213. https://doi.org/10.1016/S2589-7500(20)30077-7

Dorsey, E. R., & Ritzer, G. (2016). The McDonaldization of medicine. *JAMA Neurology*, 73(1), 15–16. https://doi.org/10.1001/jamaneurol.2015.3449

EITH ThinkTank. (2022). *Unlocking innovation to build more resilient and sustainable healthcare systems in Europe*. https://eithealth.eu/wp-content/uploads/2022/05/EITH-ThinkTank-Report_Healthcare-System-Resilience-and-Sustainability.pdf

Eit-health-and-mckinsey_transforming-healthcare-with-ai.pdf. (n.d.). Retrieved February 7, 2023, from https://eit.europa.eu/sites/default/files/eit-health-and-mckinsey_transforming-healthcare-with-ai.pdf

Eke, D. O., Chintu, S. S., & Wakunuma, K. (2023). Towards shaping the future of responsible AI in Africa. In D. O. Eke, K. Wakunuma, & S. Akintoye (Eds.), *Responsible AI in Africa:*

Challenges and opportunities (pp. 169–193). Springer International Publishing. https://doi.org/10.1007/978-3-031-08215-3_8

Esteva, A., Kuprel, B., Novoa, R. A., Ko, J., Swetter, S. M., Blau, H. M., & Thrun, S. (2017). Dermatologist-level classification of skin cancer with deep neural networks. *Nature, 542*(7639), 115–118. https://doi.org/10.1038/nature21056

Fotaki, A., Puyol-Antón, E., Chiribiri, A., Botnar, R., Pushparajah, K., & Prieto, C. (2022). Artificial intelligence in cardiac MRI: Is clinical adoption forthcoming? *Frontiers in Cardiovascular Medicine, 8*, 818765. https://doi.org/10.3389/fcvm.2021.818765

Frizzell, T. O., Glashutter, M., Liu, C. C., Zeng, A., Pan, D., Hajra, S. G., D'Arcy, R. C. N., & Song, X. (2022). Artificial intelligence in brain MRI analysis of Alzheimer's disease over the past 12 years: A systematic review. *Ageing Research Reviews, 77*, 101614. https://doi.org/10.1016/j.arr.2022.101614

Gao, Y., Dligach, D., Christensen, L., Tesch, S., Laffin, R., Xu, D., Miller, T., Uzuner, O., Churpek, M. M., & Afshar, M. (2022). A scoping review of publicly available language tasks in clinical natural language processing. *Journal of the American Medical Informatics Association, 29*(10), 1797–1806. https://doi.org/10.1093/jamia/ocac127

Gichoya, J. W., Banerjee, I., Bhimireddy, A. R., Burns, J. L., Celi, L. A., Chen, L.-C., Correa, R., Dullerud, N., Ghassemi, M., Huang, S.-C., Kuo, P.-C., Lungren, M. P., Palmer, L. J., Price, B. J., Purkayastha, S., Pyrros, A. T., Oakden-Rayner, L., Okechukwu, C., Seyyed-Kalantari, L., … Zhang, H. (2022). AI recognition of patient race in medical imaging: A modelling study. *The Lancet Digital Health, 4*(6), e406–e414. https://doi.org/10.1016/S2589-7500(22)00063-2

Gilvaz, V., Abraham, G., Radhakrishnan, S., & Hasmath, Z. (2019). From admission to discharge, how artificial intelligence could optimize patient care: A brief review. *American Journal of Hospital Medicine, 3*(4). https://doi.org/10.24150/ajhm/2019.016

Global, Regional, and Country-Specific Lifetime Risks of Stroke, 1990 and 2016. (2018). *New England Journal of Medicine, 379*(25), 2429–2437. https://doi.org/10.1056/NEJMoa1804492

Grzybowski, A., Brona, P., Lim, G., Ruamviboonsuk, P., Tan, G. S. W., Abramoff, M., & Ting, D. S. W. (2020). Artificial intelligence for diabetic retinopathy screening: A review. *Eye, 34*(3), 451–460. https://doi.org/10.1038/s41433-019-0566-0

Gulshan, V., Peng, L., Coram, M., Stumpe, M. C., Wu, D., Narayanaswamy, A., Venugopalan, S., Widner, K., Madams, T., Cuadros, J., Kim, R., Raman, R., Nelson, P. C., Mega, J. L., & Webster, D. R. (2016). Development and validation of a deep learning algorithm for detection of diabetic retinopathy in retinal fundus photographs. *JAMA, 316*(22), 2402. https://doi.org/10.1001/jama.2016.17216

Habib, A. R., Lin, A. L., & Grant, R. W. (2021). The epic sepsis model falls short—The importance of external validation. *JAMA Internal Medicine, 181*(8), 1040. https://doi.org/10.1001/jamainternmed.2021.3333

HEE-Topol-Review-2019.pdf. (n.d.). Retrieved February 10, 2023, from https://topol.hee.nhs.uk/wp-content/uploads/HEE-Topol-Review-2019.pdf

Higgins, D., & Madai, V. I. (2020). From bit to bedside: A practical framework for artificial intelligence product development in healthcare. *Advanced Intelligent Systems, 2*(10), 2000052. https://doi.org/10.1002/aisy.202000052

Hormel, T. T., Hwang, T. S., Bailey, S. T., Wilson, D. J., Huang, D., & Jia, Y. (2021). Artificial intelligence in OCT angiography. *Progress in Retinal and Eye Research, 85*, 100965. https://doi.org/10.1016/j.preteyeres.2021.100965

Idnay, B., Dreisbach, C., Weng, C., & Schnall, R. (2021). A systematic review on natural language processing systems for eligibility prescreening in clinical research. *Journal of the American Medical Informatics Association, 29*(1), 197–206. https://doi.org/10.1093/jamia/ocab228

Inui, T., Kohno, H., Kawasaki, Y., Matsuura, K., Ueda, H., Tamura, Y., Watanabe, M., Inage, Y., Yakita, Y., Wakabayashi, Y., & Matsumiya, G. (2020). Use of a smart watch for early detection of paroxysmal atrial fibrillation: Validation study. *JMIR Cardio, 4*(1), e14857. https://doi.org/10.2196/14857

Ive, J. (2022). Leveraging the potential of synthetic text for AI in mental healthcare. *Frontiers in digital health, 4*, 1010202. https://doi.org/10.3389/fdgth.2022.1010202

Ji, Z., Lee, N., Frieske, R., Yu, T., Su, D., Xu, Y., Ishii, E., Bang, Y., Madotto, A., & Fung, P. (2022). Survey of hallucination in natural language generation. *ACM Computing Surveys*, 3571730. https://doi.org/10.1145/3571730

Kelly, B. S., Judge, C., Bollard, S. M., Clifford, S. M., Healy, G. M., Aziz, A., Mathur, P., Islam, S., Yeom, K. W., Lawlor, A., & Killeen, R. P. (2022). Radiology artificial intelligence: A systematic review and evaluation of methods (RAISE). *European Radiology, 32*(11), 7998–8007. https://doi.org/10.1007/s00330-022-08784-6

Krause, J., Gulshan, V., Rahimy, E., Karth, P., Widner, K., Corrado, G. S., Peng, L., & Webster, D. R. (2018). Grader variability and the importance of reference standards for evaluating machine learning models for diabetic retinopathy. *Ophthalmology, 125*(8), 1264–1272. https://doi.org/10.1016/j.ophtha.2018.01.034

Kundeti, S. R., Vijayananda, J., Mujjiga, S., & Kalyan, M. (2016). Clinical named entity recognition: Challenges and opportunities. *2016 IEEE International Conference on Big Data (Big Data)*, 1937–1945. https://doi.org/10.1109/BigData.2016.7840814

Lambert, T. W., Smith, F., & Goldacre, M. J. (2018). Why doctors consider leaving UK medicine: Qualitative analysis of comments from questionnaire surveys three years after graduation. *Journal of the Royal Society of Medicine, 111*(1), 18–30. https://doi.org/10.1177/0141076817738502

Lee, D. Y., Kim, C., Lee, S., Son, S. J., Cho, S.-M., Cho, Y. H., Lim, J., & Park, R. W. (2022). Psychosis relapse prediction leveraging electronic health records data and natural language processing enrichment methods. *Frontiers in Psychiatry, 13*, 844442. https://doi.org/10.3389/fpsyt.2022.844442

Lee, J. M., & Hauskrecht, M. (2021). Modeling multivariate clinical event time-series with recurrent temporal mechanisms. *Artificial Intelligence in Medicine, 112*, 102021. https://doi.org/10.1016/j.artmed.2021.102021

Lemaire, J. B., & Wallace, J. E. (2017). Burnout among doctors. *BMJ, 358*, j3360. https://doi.org/10.1136/bmj.j3360

Lennox, L., Maher, L., & Reed, J. (2018). Navigating the sustainability landscape: A systematic review of sustainability approaches in healthcare. *Implementation Science, 13*(1), 27. https://doi.org/10.1186/s13012-017-0707-4

Lifetime Risk of Developing or Dying From Cancer https://www.cancer.org/cancer/cancer-basics/lifetime-probability-of-developing-or-dying-from-cancer.html. (2020). https://www.cancer.org/cancer/cancer-basics/lifetime-probability-of-developing-or-dying-from-cancer.html

Lopes, J., Guimarães, T., & Santos, M. F. (2020). Predictive and Prescriptive analytics in healthcare: A survey. *Procedia Computer Science, 170*, 1029–1034. https://doi.org/10.1016/j.procs.2020.03.078

Lorkowski, J., Maciejowska-Wilcock, I., & Pokorski, M. (2021). Overload of medical documentation: A disincentive for healthcare professionals. In M. Pokorski (Ed.), *Medical research and innovation* (pp. 1–10). Springer International Publishing. https://doi.org/10.1007/5584_2020_587

Lupu, D., Quigley, L., Mehfoud, N., & Salsberg, E. S. (2018). The growing demand for hospice and palliative medicine physicians: Will the supply keep up? *Journal of Pain and Symptom Management, 55*(4), 1216–1223. https://doi.org/10.1016/j.jpainsymman.2018.01.011

McCradden, M. D., Anderson, J. A., A. Stephenson, E., Drysdale, E., Erdman, L., Goldenberg, A., & Zlotnik Shaul, R. (2022). A research ethics framework for the clinical translation of healthcare machine learning. *The American Journal of Bioethics, 22*(5), 8–22. https://doi.org/10.1080/15265161.2021.2013977

McKay, C. (2020). Predicting risk in criminal procedure: Actuarial tools, algorithms, AI and judicial decision-making. *Current Issues in Criminal Justice, 32*(1), 22–39. https://doi.org/10.1080/10345329.2019.1658694

Mellouli, T., & Stoeck, T. (2021). AI/OR synergies of process mining with optimal planning of patient pathways for effective hospital-wide decision support. In M. Masmoudi, B. Jarboui, & P. Siarry (Eds.), *Artificial intelligence and data mining in healthcare* (pp. 23–54). Springer International Publishing. https://doi.org/10.1007/978-3-030-45240-7_2

Mikolov, T., Chen, K., Corrado, G., & Dean, J. (2013). *Efficient estimation of word representations in vector space*. https://doi.org/10.48550/ARXIV.1301.3781

Muehlematter, U. J., Daniore, P., & Vokinger, K. N. (2021). Approval of artificial intelligence and machine learning-based medical devices in the USA and Europe (2015–20): A comparative analysis. *The Lancet Digital Health*, 3(3), e195–e203. https://doi.org/10.1016/S2589-7500(20)30292-2

Munavalli, J. R., Boersma, H. J., Rao, S. V., & van Merode, G. G. (2021). Real-time capacity management and patient flow optimization in hospitals using AI methods. In M. Masmoudi, B. Jarboui, & P. Siarry (Eds.), *Artificial intelligence and data mining in healthcare* (pp. 55–69). Springer International Publishing. https://doi.org/10.1007/978-3-030-45240-7_3

Nelson, A., Herron, D., Rees, G., & Nachev, P. (2019). Predicting scheduled hospital attendance with artificial intelligence. *NPJ Digital Medicine*, 2(1), Article 1. https://doi.org/10.1038/s41746-019-0103-3

Noncommunicable diseases. (n.d.). Retrieved November 27, 2022, from https://www.who.int/health-topics/noncommunicable-diseases

Norori, N., Hu, Q., Aellen, F. M., Faraci, F. D., & Tzovara, A. (2021). Addressing bias in big data and AI for health care: A call for open science. *Patterns*, 2(10), 100347. https://doi.org/10.1016/j.patter.2021.100347

Noseworthy, J., Madara, J., Cosgrove, D., Edgeworth, M., Ellison, E., Krevans, S., Rothman, P., Sowers, K., Strongwater, S., Torchiana, D., & Harrison, D. (n.d.). Physician burnout is a public health crisis: A message to our fellow health care CEOs. *Health Affairs Forefront*. https://doi.org/10.1377/forefront.20170328.059397

OECD. (2015). *Fiscal sustainability of health systems: Bridging health and finance perspectives.* Organisation for Economic Co-operation and Development. https://www.oecd-ilibrary.org/social-issues-migration-health/fiscal-sustainability-of-health-systems_9789264233386-en

OECD. (2017). *Tackling wasteful spending on health.* Organisation for Economic Co-operation and Development. https://www.oecd-ilibrary.org/social-issues-migration-health/tackling-wasteful-spending-on-health_9789264266414-en

Owoyemi, A., Owoyemi, J., Osiyemi, A., & Boyd, A. (2020). Artificial intelligence for healthcare in Africa. *Frontiers in Digital Health*, 2. https://www.frontiersin.org/articles/10.3389/fdgth.2020.00006

Panch, T., Mattie, H., & Celi, L. A. (2019). The "inconvenient truth" about AI in healthcare. *NPJ Digital Medicine*, 2(1), 77. https://doi.org/10.1038/s41746-019-0155-4

Parekh, D., Poddar, N., Rajpurkar, A., Chahal, M., Kumar, N., Joshi, G. P., & Cho, W. (2022). A review on autonomous vehicles: Progress, methods and challenges. *Electronics*, 11(14), Article 14. https://doi.org/10.3390/electronics11142162

Phan, T. G., Haseeb, A., Beare, R., Srikanth, V., Thrift, A. G., & Ma, H. (2020). Googling the lifetime risk of stroke around the world. *Frontiers in Neurology*, 11. https://www.frontiersin.org/articles/10.3389/fneur.2020.00729

Qader, W. A., Ameen, M. M., & Ahmed, B. I. (2019). An overview of bag of words; importance, implementation, applications, and challenges. *2019 International Engineering Conference (IEC)*, 200–204. https://doi.org/10.1109/IEC47844.2019.8950616

Qin, Y., Kernan, K. F., Fan, Z., Park, H.-J., Kim, S., Canna, S. W., Kellum, J. A., Berg, R. A., Wessel, D., Pollack, M. M., Meert, K., Hall, M., Newth, C., Lin, J. C., Doctor, A., Shanley, T., Cornell, T., Harrison, R. E., Zuppa, A. F., … Carcillo, J. A. (2022). Machine learning derivation of four computable 24-h pediatric sepsis phenotypes to facilitate enrollment in early personalized anti-inflammatory clinical trials. *Critical Care*, 26(1), 128. https://doi.org/10.1186/s13054-022-03977-3

Rajpurkar, P., Chen, E., Banerjee, O., & Topol, E. J. (2022). AI in health and medicine. *Nature Medicine*, *28*(1), 31–38. https://doi.org/10.1038/s41591-021-01614-0

Rea, F., Corrao, G., Ludergnani, M., Cajazzo, L., & Merlino, L. (2019). A new population-based risk stratification tool was developed and validated for predicting mortality, hospital admissions, and health care costs. *Journal of Clinical Epidemiology*, *116*, 62–71. https://doi.org/10.1016/j.jclinepi.2019.08.009

Reddy, S. (2022). Explainability and artificial intelligence in medicine. *The Lancet Digital Health*, *4*(4), e214–e215. https://doi.org/10.1016/S2589-7500(22)00029-2

Reddy, S., Fox, J., & Purohit, M. P. (2019). Artificial intelligence-enabled healthcare delivery. *Journal of the Royal Society of Medicine*, *112*(1), 22–28. https://doi.org/10.1177/0141076818815510

Reuter-Oppermann, M., & Kühl, N. (2021). Artificial intelligence for healthcare logistics: An overview and research agenda. In M. Masmoudi, B. Jarboui, & P. Siarry (Eds.), *Artificial intelligence and data mining in healthcare* (pp. 1–22). Springer International Publishing. https://doi.org/10.1007/978-3-030-45240-7_1

Rimmer, A. (2017). The UK needs more generalists, but where will they come from? *BMJ*, *356*, j1116. https://doi.org/10.1136/bmj.j1116

Romero-Brufau, S., Whitford, D., Johnson, M. G., Hickman, J., Morlan, B. W., Therneau, T., Naessens, J., & Huddleston, J. M. (2021). Using machine learning to improve the accuracy of patient deterioration predictions: Mayo clinic early warning score (MC-EWS). *Journal of the American Medical Informatics Association*, *28*(6), 1207–1215. https://doi.org/10.1093/jamia/ocaa347

Russakovsky, O., Deng, J., Su, H., Krause, J., Satheesh, S., Ma, S., Huang, Z., Karpathy, A., Khosla, A., Bernstein, M., Berg, A. C., & Fei-Fei, L. (2015). ImageNet large scale visual recognition challenge. *International Journal of Computer Vision*, *115*(3), 211–252. https://doi.org/10.1007/s11263-015-0816-y

Sahni, N., Stein, G., Zemmel, R., & Cutler, D. M. (2023). *The potential impact of artificial intelligence on healthcare spending* (Working Paper No. 30857). National Bureau of Economic Research. https://doi.org/10.3386/w30857

Scheffler, R. M., & Arnold, D. R. (2019). Projecting shortages and surpluses of doctors and nurses in the OECD: What looms ahead. *Health Economics, Policy and Law*, *14*(2), 274–290. https://doi.org/10.1017/S174413311700055X

Seah, J. C. Y., Tang, C. H. M., Buchlak, Q. D., Holt, X. G., Wardman, J. B., Aimoldin, A., Esmaili, N., Ahmad, H., Pham, H., Lambert, J. F., Hachey, B., Hogg, S. J. F., Johnston, B. P., Bennett, C., Oakden-Rayner, L., Brotchie, P., & Jones, C. M. (2021). Effect of a comprehensive deep-learning model on the accuracy of chest x-ray interpretation by radiologists: A retrospective, multireader multicase study. *The Lancet Digital Health*, *3*(8), e496–e506. https://doi.org/10.1016/S2589-7500(21)00106-0

Searle, T., Ibrahim, Z., Teo, J., & Dobson, R. (2022). *Summarisation of electronic health records with clinical concept guidance*. https://doi.org/10.48550/ARXIV.2211.07126

Sengupta, E., Jain, N., Garg, D., & Choudhury, T. (2018). A review of payment card fraud detection methods using artificial intelligence. *2018 International Conference on Computational Techniques, Electronics and Mechanical Systems (CTEMS)*, 494–498. https://doi.org/10.1109/CTEMS.2018.8769160

Shwartz-Ziv, R., & Armon, A. (2021). *Tabular data: Deep learning is not all you need*. https://doi.org/10.48550/ARXIV.2106.03253

Sipari, D., Chaparro-Rico, B. D. M., & Cafolla, D. (2022). SANE (Easy Gait Analysis System): Towards an AI-assisted automatic gait-analysis. *International Journal of Environmental Research and Public Health*, *19*(16), 10032. https://doi.org/10.3390/ijerph191610032

Teo, J. T. H., Dinu, V., Bernal, W., Davidson, P., Oliynyk, V., Breen, C., Barker, R. D., & Dobson, R. J. B. (2021). Real-time clinician text feeds from electronic health records. *NPJ Digital Medicine*, *4*(1), 35. https://doi.org/10.1038/s41746-021-00406-7

The INFORM-lab, Palmer, E., Klapaukh, R., Harris, S., & Singer, M. (2019). Intelligently learning from data. *Critical Care*, 23(1). https://doi.org/10.1186/s13054-019-2424-7

Tilmes, N. (2022). Disability, fairness, and algorithmic bias in AI recruitment. *Ethics and Information Technology*, 24(2), 21. https://doi.org/10.1007/s10676-022-09633-2

Topol, E. J. (2019). High-performance medicine: The convergence of human and artificial intelligence. *Nature Medicine*, 25(1), 44–56. https://doi.org/10.1038/s41591-018-0300-7

Tsui, F. R., Shi, L., Ruiz, V., Ryan, N. D., Biernesser, C., Iyengar, S., Walsh, C. G., & Brent, D. A. (2021). Natural language processing and machine learning of electronic health records for prediction of first-time suicide attempts. *JAMIA Open*, 4(1), ooab011. https://doi.org/10.1093/jamiaopen/ooab011

Voelker, R. (2020). Cardiac ultrasound uses artificial intelligence to produce images. *JAMA*, 323(11), 1034. https://doi.org/10.1001/jama.2020.2547

WEF_PHSSR_Interim_Report_of_the_Pilot_Phase.pdf. (n.d.). Retrieved February 7, 2023, from https://www3.weforum.org/docs/WEF_PHSSR_Interim_Report_of_the_Pilot_Phase.pdf

West, C. P., Tan, A. D., Habermann, T. M., Sloan, J. A., & Shanafelt, T. D. (2009). Association of resident fatigue and distress with perceived medical errors. *JAMA*, 302(12), 1294–1300. https://doi.org/10.1001/jama.2009.1389

Whang, S. E., Roh, Y., Song, H., & Lee, J.-G. (2021). *Data collection and quality challenges in deep learning: A data-centric AI perspective*. https://doi.org/10.48550/ARXIV.2112.06409

Whebell, S., & Zhang, J. (2022). Bringing biological ARDS phenotypes to the bedside with machine-learning-based classifiers. *The Lancet Respiratory Medicine*, 10(4), 319–320. https://doi.org/10.1016/S2213-2600(21)00492-6

Wong, A., Otles, E., Donnelly, J. P., Krumm, A., McCullough, J., DeTroyer-Cooley, O., Pestrue, J., Phillips, M., Konye, J., Penoza, C., Ghous, M., & Singh, K. (2021). External validation of a widely implemented proprietary sepsis prediction model in hospitalized patients. *JAMA Internal Medicine*, 181(8), 1065. https://doi.org/10.1001/jamainternmed.2021.2626

World Health Organization. (2007). *Everybody's business -- strengthening health systems to improve health outcomes: WHO's framework for action*. 44.

World Health Organization = Organisation mondiale de la Santé. (2007). Health systems for health security – Strengthening prevention, preparedness and response to health emergencies. *Weekly Epidemiological Record = Relevé Épidémiologique Hebdomadaire*, 96(19), 157–163.

World Population Prospects 2022: Summary of Results. (n.d.). 52.

Wu, S., Roberts, K., Datta, S., Du, J., Ji, Z., Si, Y., Soni, S., Wang, Q., Wei, Q., Xiang, Y., Zhao, B., & Xu, H. (2020). Deep learning in clinical natural language processing: A methodical review. *Journal of the American Medical Informatics Association*, 27(3), 457–470. https://doi.org/10.1093/jamia/ocz200

Yamashita, R., Nishio, M., Do, R. K. G., & Togashi, K. (2018). Convolutional neural networks: An overview and application in radiology. *Insights into Imaging*, 9(4), 611–629. https://doi.org/10.1007/s13244-018-0639-9

Yang, X., Bian, J., Hogan, W. R., & Wu, Y. (2020). Clinical concept extraction using transformers. *Journal of the American Medical Informatics Association*, 27(12), 1935–1942. https://doi.org/10.1093/jamia/ocaa189

Yu, S. C., Shivakumar, N., Betthauser, K., Gupta, A., Lai, A. M., Kollef, M. H., Payne, P. R. O., & Michelson, A. P. (2021). Comparison of early warning scores for sepsis early identification and prediction in the general ward setting. *JAMIA Open*, 4(3), ooab062. https://doi.org/10.1093/jamiaopen/ooab062

Zhang, J., Budhdeo, S., William, W., Cerrato, P., Shuaib, H., Sood, H., Ashrafian, H., Halamka, J., & Teo, J. T. (2022a). Moving towards vertically integrated artificial intelligence development. *NPJ Digital Medicine*, 5(1), 143. https://doi.org/10.1038/s41746-022-00690-x

Zhang, J., Mattie, H., Shuaib, H., Hensman, T., Teo, J. T., & Celi, L. A. (2022b). Addressing the "elephant in the room" of AI clinical decision support through organisation-level regulation. *PLOS Digital Health*, 1(9), e0000111. https://doi.org/10.1371/journal.pdig.0000111

Zhang, J., Symons, J., Agapow, P., Teo, J. T., Paxton, C. A., Abdi, J., Mattie, H., Davie, C., Torres, A. Z., Folarin, A., Sood, H., Celi, L. A., Halamka, J., Eapen, S., & Budhdeo, S. (2022c). Best practices in the real-world data life cycle. *PLOS Digital Health*, 1(1), e0000003. https://doi.org/10.1371/journal.pdig.0000003

Zhang, J., Whebell, S., Gallifant, J., Budhdeo, S., Mattie, H., Lertvittayakumjorn, P., del Pilar Arias Lopez, M., Tiangco, B. J., Gichoya, J. W., Ashrafian, H., Celi, L. A., & Teo, J. T. (2022d). An interactive dashboard to track themes, development maturity, and global equity in clinical artificial intelligence research. *The Lancet Digital Health*, 4(4), e212–e213. https://doi.org/10.1016/S2589-7500(22)00032-2

Zhang, J., Whebell, S. F., Sanderson, B., Retter, A., Daly, K., Paul, R., Barrett, N., Agarwal, S., Lams, B. E., Meadows, C., Terblanche, M., & Camporota, L. (2021). Phenotypes of severe COVID-19 ARDS receiving extracorporeal membrane oxygenation. *British Journal of Anaesthesia*, 126(3), e130–e132. https://doi.org/10.1016/j.bja.2020.12.023

4

Technical Issues in Implementing AI in Healthcare

Sonika Tyagi

RMIT, Melbourne, Australia

LEARNING OBJECTIVES

- Describe the role of AI in healthcare and what it aims to accomplish.
- Discuss the technical challenges in implementing AI in healthcare settings.
- Discuss the algorithmic challenges of developing actionable outcomes and AI for social good.
- Describe approaches to tackle some of the challenges.

Introduction

In recent years, Artificial Intelligence (AI) has led to breakthroughs in several areas, and it is transforming our daily lives completely. AI can play and beat the best human players in chess, drive cars and even make music and write poems. But what about healthcare? The application of AI in healthcare are not merely a future possibility. It has indeed become a present clinical reality, and even organizations such as the Food and Drug Administration (FDA) approve of autonomous artificial intelligence diagnostic systems (Mesko, 2019; Topol, 2019). There are several reasons why we are all excited about the trajectory we are all on in AI and healthcare.

AI can not only save lives and improve care for millions of patients around the world, but it is also helping us personalize the delivery of care, making hospitals more efficient, and improving access to healthcare by providing accurate decision-making tools (Matheny et al., 2020). Machine learning (ML), a subset of AI, has been the most popular approach of current AI healthcare applications in recent times since it allows computational systems to learn from data and improve their performance without being explicitly programmed. ML algorithms learn from large and complex datasets through a process known as 'training' to build 'models' that can be used to make decisions or predict outcomes. For instance, a computer algorithm can learn from the data of thousands of patients whether or not a treatment is going to work, and what works best for an individual based on their individual conditions. The European Union (EU) has predicted that adaptation of AI in healthcare can change 400,000 lives, 200 billion Euros and 1.8 billion hours annually in the EU alone (Eliana Biundo et al., 2020), and we may expect similar

DOI: 10.1201/9781003262152-4

trends of socioeconomic impact on the global scale. Similarly, AI in healthcare market is expected to experience significant growth with prediction going from USD14.6 billion in 2023 to USD102.7 billion by 2028 (Vishal & Onkar, 2021).

Electronic medical records (EMR) are being used to create AI that can help uncover clinical best practices and analyse clinical practice trends acquired from EMR to develop new clinical practice models. Similarly, the future of drug discovery and the development process is expected to be simplified and accelerated using AI. AI can convert a labour-intensive drug discovery process to a data-intensive one by using robotics, models of genetics, drugs, diseases, and their progression, along with pharmacokinetics, safety, and efficacy characteristics. AI-driven drug discovery is likely to be fast and more cost-effective. Although, just as with the development of a new drug, the identification of a lead molecule does not guarantee a successful therapy and requires more downstream validations. The scope of emerging AI-driven healthcare applications is very broad in terms of their objectives and creation and how and where they might be used. These applications range from entirely self-sufficient robotic surgery to non-self-sufficient mortality forecasts or the length of hospital stay and the estimations of resource allocation (Schwalbe & Wahl, 2020).

Challenges and Limitations of AI Adoption in Healthcare

There is no question that AI will be a dramatic component of healthcare and in the future, we won't believe how we did certain tasks in the past without using AI. The question to consider at this point is: Will it be safe? Can we trust it? Have you ever wondered how it would be to be treated by AI instead of a human doctor? Here, we are not talking about turning our healthcare over to computers and robots. Instead, we are talking about augmenting the routine tasks of humans. As an example, a radiologist that diagnoses medical imaging would be replaced by a radiologist that would use AI tools. A radiologist may be performing hundreds of highly complex tasks every day; not only diagnosing images but also planning scan procedures, informing patients, and even performing interventions. Therefore, you need to provide hundreds of AI tools, one for each of those tasks that they perform to replace a single radiologist. It is now understandable that healthcare physicians, medical scientists and patients will be using these AI tools. Healthcare professionals can amplify what they routinely do as humans and spend more time with patients, increasing the overall efficiency of the system.

There are numerous factors that are slowing the adoption of AI in healthcare settings. One category of the technical challenges includes complexities and limitations inherent to machine learning algorithms and their implementation (Figure 4.1). We understand that AI can carry out very narrow predefined tasks. Even though AI can beat the best human players in chess, it can do absolutely nothing else at all. In the overwhelming majority of present-day references to AI, we mean machines that can learn. However, machines are very bad at learning stuff, at least when compared to humans. Taking an example of learning to distinguish between pictures of two animals. Humans can learn it quickly with quite a low error rate. But in the case of ML, you must use the best of algorithms, which will require thousands of images to learn and still may not achieve the same low error rates as humans.

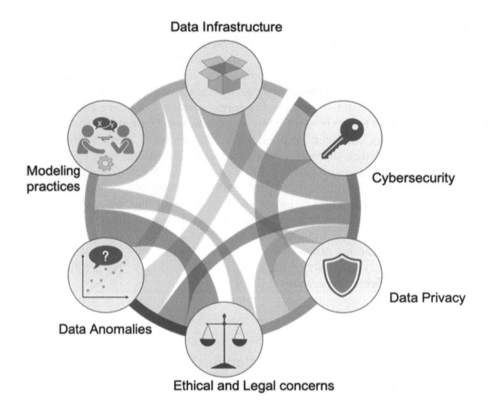

FIGURE 4.1
Key technical challenges in applying AI in healthcare.

(Source: illustration prepared with assistance from Tyrone Chen of Monash University.)

The artificial neural network (ANN) algorithms are a popular choice of ML algorithm which is loosely based on how neurons connect in the human brain to pass information. The major challenge here is that these algorithms are so-called black boxes. Because we don't understand at a deep level how these algorithms arrive at a decision or outcome prediction, at least not in a human-intelligible way. Why should a doctor trust the output of a system without knowing why the algorithm predicts something and if it cannot provide the reasoning for its decision, which has an impact on human lives? Even though techniques exist to open these black boxes, they are not perfect and thus pose a huge challenge in healthcare. Describing how those outputs can be included in the research, along with predictions can help assess the cost of the scientific trial and guide scientific research.

There are not only the AI-specific reasons that pose hurdles in the way of adoption of AI in healthcare; there are also healthcare-specific reasons. Healthcare is a complex system made of hospitals, physicians, clinicians, ER etc. it is neither simple, nor desirable, nor even possible to completely disrupt such a system. The change is not possible overnight; it must be gradual. One of many ways would be to augment healthcare tasks with technology along with education and awareness of the downstream benefits of potential transformations.

The third category of challenges in deploying AI in healthcare is its regulation. For instance, we have created a medical device that needs to be certified according to the regulatory laws of our region. Either such law may not already exist or to develop tools according to these requirements that fulfil them may take many years.

Some of these challenges will be discussed in more detail below.

Data Infrastructure

Data infrastructures refer to data storage, access, standardization, and data protection (Lindley et al., 2020). Healthcare data comes in various shapes and sizes and is generally stored either as relational databases or via authorized data registries and data containers. The sensitive data contains personal health information (PHI) that would enable a researcher to identify a participant. Therefore, the access to data involves ethics approval and a protected environment with the highest standards for privacy, confidentiality, and data security for computing purposes. To conduct sophisticated data analysis for health informatics the compute infrastructure requirement goes beyond personal computers and hard drives. Secure clouds are becoming a commonly used data infrastructure. Clouds supports more flexible work and business operations such that larger volumes of data can be stored and accessed more readily. However, it may also require specialized skills to set up and use clouds efficiently. Further, different data pre-processing techniques are used to select, store, prepare, enhance, and share the data appropriately. Although usage of data from a single site is common in retrospective clinical studies, it is getting increasingly difficult to perform open research due to patient privacy concerns and efforts involved in de-identifying it. Moreover, the results obtained from single-site data are difficult to generalize due to a lack of diversity. It is also difficult to judge one method from another if they are not obtained from the same underlying data. However, to integrate data from multiple sites requires adoption of common data models such as OMOP [https://ohdsi.org/omop/] or data exchange formats, such as FHIR (Duda et al., 2022) and HL7 standards [https://www.hl7.org/] that would again require awareness and skills to deploy such standards. Similarly, applying controlled data vocabularies [https://guides.lib.umich.edu/ontology/ontologies] would enhance data integration, interoperability, and scalability of such data infrastructures [https://www.himss.org/resources/interoperability-healthcare].

Training AI tools on poor-quality data is one of the most common problems in healthcare. This is because of the limited access to data that does not accurately represent its underlying real-world mechanisms. Adopting common standards for data sharing and access can help alleviate these issues. On the other hand, obtaining high-quality data is another major challenge. In the case of medical imaging a single model may require thousands of images; pre-processing and annotating these files is a time-consuming and expensive process, even when automated.

Data Privacy

When it comes to the healthcare industry, privacy is a prominent issue. Patient data contains highly sensitive PHI (e.g., medical histories, identity information, payment information), which is protected by regulations such as General Data Protection and Regulation (GDPR) and Health Insurance Portability and Accountability Act (HIPAA).

The GDPR, in particular, aims to protect the right of natural persons to the protection of personal data [Art. 1(2) of the GDPR]. While the HIPAA Privacy Rule (45 C.F.R. Part 160; A and E of Part 164) is the key federal law to protect health data privacy.

In addition, the AI algorithms are very data-hungry in the process of learning from data. We do have a large amount of data available from studies, registries, and from electronic medical records (EMR) but we can't use all this data due to data privacy laws and also due to the fact it's hard to properly anonymize data. Operational silos in health informatics hinder ability to utilize data for new research development and innovations. Hence, policy makers globally are considering it as their primary priority to extend healthcare delivery beyond the healthcare facility. At the technical level various data encryption methods, such as data masking or anonymization, have been proposed to ensure multi-level privacy. These techniques replace sensitive data with fictitious or obfuscated values in non-production environments. This reduces the risk of exposing real sensitive data during development or testing. Other strategies include the concept of cryptography along with statistical modelling (Yang et al., 2015), third party solutions using Public Key Encryption (PKE) and Diffe-Hellman key exchanges (Wang et al., 2014), and Wireless Sensor Network (WSN) cloud-based solutions that uses Attribute Based Encryption (ABE) and Symmetric Key Cryptography (SKC) (Lounis et al., 2016).

Conducting regular security audits and vulnerability assessments to identify any weaknesses or potential security breaches can mitigate some these challenges. This includes both internal audits performed by your organization and external audits conducted by third-party security experts.

Cybersecurity

Due to the sensitivity of personal health data, AI systems can become prone to data breaches and identity theft. Criminals can use AI to cause system malfunction or gain access to systems without permission. Additionally, as AI becomes smarter and able to make autonomous decisions, it will be able to execute automated cyberattacks without human intervention. Thus, the cybersecurity issue is one of the biggest challenges in AI technology. The large data requirements of most AI models and concerns over the possibility of data leakages also reduce the adoption of healthcare AI technologies (Nguyen et al., 2022). Creating a highly secure infrastructure to gather and store the data generated is paramount in tackling these challenges (Ghafur et al., 2019). To resolve this issue, one can begin by identifying and classifying the sensitive data within a system. Determine which data needs higher levels of protection based on its confidentiality, integrity, and availability requirements. Secondly, one can implement strict access controls to ensure that sensitive data is only accessible to authorized individuals or systems. This can be achieved through techniques such as role-based access control (RBAC), where access privileges are assigned based on users' roles and responsibilities. Techniques such as homomorphic encryption (Wood et al., 2020) are being used to keep information private and secure even while sending them over a network. Isolating the system containing sensitive data from other networks, especially those that are publicly accessible or less secure is desirable here. Further, implementation of firewalls, intrusion detection systems, and other network security measures to monitor and control access to the system is recommended.

Federated learning (FL), where AI models are trained collaboratively on the edge, is another upcoming solution which is different to the traditional approach of training models on data gathered in one place or assuming that data is identically distributed (Nguyen et al., 2022). The FL way of decentralized approach enables multiple algorithms to build a common, robust AI model without exchanging data thus allowing to avoid issues of data privacy and security. These new AI models can train on data that never leaves your mobile phone, laptop, or a private server allowing to address critical issues of access to heterogeneous and sensitive data.

Ethical and Legal Concerns

The rise of AI in high-risk situations has increased the requirement for accountable, equitable, and transparent AI design and governance (Naik et al., 2022). Common ethical challenges refer to (1) informed consent to use, (2) safety and transparency, (3) algorithmic fairness and biases, and (4) data privacy, that we have discussed in the previous sections. Whereas *legal* challenges generally involve (1) safety and effectiveness, (2) liability, (3) data protection and privacy, (4) cybersecurity, and (5) intellectual property law (Gerke et al., 2020).

Data Anomalies

From a research perspective, healthcare data poses numerous challenges. Among the most common ones are heterogeneity, missingness, medical errors, censored data, irregularity, fragmentations, and biases (Shah & Khan, 2020). The "missingness" can be caused due to the failure to record a measurement, non-availability of data, or technical issues. Fragmentation of the data and the mismatch occurring due to lack of interoperability between different sources through which the data is being originally recorded. Healthcare data is episodic in nature, made up of intermittent measurements scattered over with varying gaps between them, making the data irregular. A main characteristic of ML is that it is a data-driven method meaning that we don't need to specifically program what to learn, instead we provide the data that contains the input and also contains the output that we want to predict. The learning process will come up with a software model that can predict for us. As a data-driven approach ML will learn from data as is, even if the data contains bias and other problems i.e. if your data contains bias the resulting model will contain that bias. This is a big challenge in healthcare. It has been known for decades that much of the medical data is heavily biased. It may often be representative of a certain population or ethnicity (Obermeyer et al., 2019). Since the level of fairness of an AI system depends on the data they are trained on and how the algorithms define what is "good" or "bad", with biased data and algorithms, the entire system could become flawed and lead to unethical and unfair results. 'Bad' data is often associated with, ethnic, communal, gender or racial biases.

Modelling Practices

Data modelling best practices in the ML domain would fall into the following three categories: 1) Data: Understanding the data that will be used to support the goals of an experiment and to consider any limitations of the data that need to be addressed. Exploratory data analysis (EDA) can help get insight into the data anomalies and pre-process them to prepare high-quality data prior to performing any ML tasks on them. Independent tests on assessing quality and quantity of data can help save time and enhance the quality of the models built on them. 2) ML modelling: Care must be taken when choosing appropriate models, ensuring enough data and correct splits to perform training, validation, and tests. Feature selection and hyperparameter tuning to optimize best settings are keys to generate robust generalizable models. This is also worth thinking about how the models will be deployed in a real-world situation. 3) Validation strategies: How the true performance of models will be measured in a meaningful and informative way should be part of the study design itself (Ozaydin et al., 2021). Testing models under various conditions, reporting multiple performance metrics, and cross-validating multiple times provides deep insight into the performance or models and their limitations. This not only increases robustness and transparencies of the models but also builds trust in the users that will be using them in real-life scenarios (Futoma et al., 2020; Prosperi et al., 2020).

CASE STUDY 1:   IMPORTANCE OF MODELLING PRACTICES

In 2012, doctors at Memorial Sloan Kettering Cancer Centre partnered with IBM to train their supercomputer Watson to diagnose and treat patients. It was a conglomeration of IBM with companies like Truven, Phytel, Explorys merging Truven's biggest insurance database in the nation contained 300 million records. Whereas Explorys and Phytel provided access to electronic health records representing over 50 million patients, and Merge contributed an extensive imaging database to the collaboration. The idea was to use all this data with Watson to find patterns amongst the high volume or variables that physicians and analysts otherwise possibly couldn't see.

However, later Watson for Oncology came under fire for allegedly not delivering on expectations to provide state-of-the-art personalized treatment for patients with cancer. The underlying AI algorithms were criticized for producing advice that is "unsafe and incorrect" (Gerke et al., 2020). This was found to be a problem with the training and testing strategies of the model, which meant that the software was only trained on "synthetic" cancer cases. It was also confirmed that these anomalies were detected during the testing phase of the system and that no real recommendations were provided to the patients. This incident put the field in a bad light and also highlights the importance of ethical, transparent, and reliable AI practices that address biases in the data and algorithms through a continuous check of the validity of the datasets (Ozaydin et al., 2021).

Moving forward, the idea of using technologies such as IBM Watson and large volumes of linked data hold promise not only for holistic patient care at the lowest possible cost but also in terms of saving lives and healthcare resources alike (Tong et al., 2022). Millions die of cancer and chronic illness each year. This rate can be slowed down through screening and preventions and by ensuring early diagnosis and state-of-the-art care. AI can gather evidence from literature and highly heterogeneous individual-specific data to help physicians make informed decisions and thus provide clinical decision support AI can also be used to increase clinical trial participation and success by identifying appropriate individuals for a clinical study. This would require going through a high number of factors from demographic information, eligibility criteria and clinical guidelines to marry up information and finding suitable candidates with a quick turnaround time. The excitement to leverage technology to support high-quality patient care remains and tech companies continue to work on the audacious health challenges with several successful outcomes.

Despite the technical issues raised earlier in the chapter, the healthcare industry is experiencing a significant transformation driven by AI innovations that are revolutionizing the way we deliver medical services. These ground-breaking advancements are disrupting traditional healthcare practices and reshaping the future of patient care. With these transformative AI innovations, the future of healthcare is poised for unprecedented advancements and improved patient outcomes. Some areas of applied AI in healthcare are recounted here.

1. **Healthcare administration**: AI-powered health administration can help reduce routine, error-prone manual tasks, save costs, and reduce fraud for insurers, payers and providers alike.

2. **Digital therapeutics (DTx)**: DTx involves leveraging evidence-based digital intervention in addition to medications and prescriptions. This is done through digital devices, including smartphone applications and wearable sensors, that can provide treatment if the evidence is valid. Healthcare providers can monitor patient progress more efficiently and provide more tailored treatments. DTx solutions are becoming increasingly popular due to both their effectiveness and affordability. Studies have suggested that DTx can be more cost-effective and that they may have fewer side effects than standard treatments. They are used to treat or manage a variety of conditions, including chronic pain, depression, allergies, anxiety, and sleep disorders.

3. **Virtual clinics**: Using a combination of ML, biosensors and telecommunication technologies, patients can be monitored virtually anywhere in the world. This reduces uncomfortable hospital visits, long wait times, and the possibility of catching another illness due to proximity to a source. This can also provide the real-time analysis of data while patients are in the comfort of their homes.

4. **Robotic surgeries**: Intertwining AI and robotics is a logical step. As clinical trials continue to demonstrate, the safety and efficacy of utilizing robots in surgery and other medical procedures, AI is being applied to further enhance their speed and accuracy while making delicate incisions. This also reduces the issue of fatigue of healthcare professionals during long and crucial procedures.

5. **Chatbots**: AI software conducting conversation via auditory or textual methods can engage users through chatrooms or other messaging services. The chatbot trend is on the rise in healthcare. These are designed to assist patients by

keeping them informed while they wait for appointments or treatments; they can also provide 24/7 accessibility to medical assistance.

6. **Patient-centred care**: AI allows to link various kinds of health and lifestyle information for an individual, thus learning a 360-degree view of the patient. AI-powered diagnosis and treatment plans serve as a third-party perspective that can lead to a better understanding between carer and patient, thereby enhancing the chances of a better outcome in the end and also even boosting patient engagement. AI tools, such as wearables and customized medical gadgets, can also be used to increase patient engagement and compliance. Non-compliance generally hinders the expected health outcomes as patients don't take initiatives to take prescriptions as directed.

7. **Research and Training**: Data-driven research using AI tools is already making a big impact in research with tools already available to predict the risk for various cancers, analysing thousands of images quickly to find informative patterns or predicting biomolecules that can be biomarkers for therapies. Similarly, AI-powered tools are being used to simulate teaching environments, involving virtual patients, preparing synthetic datasets or even AI-tutors such as ChatGPT can help with learning.

8. **Drug discovery**: Pharmaceutical companies that use vast datasets to identify patient response to develop viable drug targets can now reap the benefits of AI by significantly cutting costs and time to market a new drug.

9. **Affordable healthcare**: AI is enabling personalized care and treatment which will eventually reduce the cost both to the patients and to the care providers by identifying the risks in advance and preparing and optimizing healthcare resources accordingly.

10. **Tech giants in primary care**: Nearly all big-tech giant companies are taking up the audacious challenge of solving complex health problems. This is a win–win situation for both the digital health workers and tech companies as we collaborate to solve complex tasks.

SUMMARY

Applications of AI in healthcare have become a present clinical reality with several autonomous AI diagnostic systems being developed and used.

A comprehensive intelligent platform that automates tedious clinical tasks would allow providers more time for their patients.

AI is transforming the healthcare system to become more patient-focused and the one that can provide holistic care and personalized treatments.

Although digital health is benefitting from the advanced applications of ML and AI, the adoption of AI in healthcare settings still faces several challenges.

Both awareness and transparency are needed for accounting potential bias in data and algorithms and building trust with all stakeholders involved.

We require global ethical frameworks around sensitive data sharing and the regulation of AI such that a greater part of society can benefit from it equitably.

REVIEW QUESTIONS

What are the main concerns of data sharing and security in digital health?

What are some of the key points setting up a digital data infrastructure to ensure reliability and scalability?

How would you design an AI-driven digital therapeutic system? What would be some of the salient features and key challenges to overcome?

Why do you think the major tech providers are making their way into primary care?

What does "AI for social good" mean to you?

References

Duda, S. N., Kennedy, N., Conway, D., Cheng, A. C., Nguyen, V., Zayas-Cabán, T., & Harris, P. A. (2022). HL7 FHIR-based tools and initiatives to support clinical research: A scoping review. *Journal of the American Medical Informatics Association, 29*(9), 1642–1653. https://doi.org/10.1093/jamia/ocac105

Eliana, Biundo, Andrew, Pease, Koen, Segers, Michael, de Groote, Thibault, D'Argent, & Schaetzen, E. D. (2020). *The socio-economic impact of AI in healthcare.* https://www.medtecheurope.org/wp-content/uploads/2020/10/mte-ai_impact-in-healthcare_oct2020_report.pdf

Futoma, J., Simons, M., Panch, T., Doshi-Velez, F., & Celi, L. A. (2020, September 01). The myth of generalisability in clinical research and machine learning in health care. *The Lancet Digital Health, 2*(9), e489–e492. https://doi.org/10.1016/S2589-7500(20)30186-2

Gerke, S., Minssen, T., & Cohen, G. (2020). Chapter 12 – Ethical and legal challenges of artificial intelligence-driven healthcare. In A. Bohr & K. Memarzadeh (Eds.), *Artificial intelligence in healthcare* (pp. 295–336). Academic Press. https://doi.org/10.1016/B978-0-12-818438-7.00012-5

Ghafur, S., Grass, E., Jennings, N. R., & Darzi, A. (2019, 05 01). The challenges of cybersecurity in health care: The UK National health service as a case study. *The Lancet Digital Health, 1*(1), e10–e12. https://doi.org/10.1016/S2589-7500(19)30005-6

Lindley, L. C., Svynarenko, R., & Profant, T. L. (2020). Data infrastructure for sensitive data: Nursing's role in the development of a secure research enclave. *CIN: Computers, Informatics, Nursing, 38*(9). https://journals.lww.com/cinjournal/Fulltext/2020/09000/Data_Infrastructure_for_Sensitive_Data__Nursing_s.1.aspx

Lounis, A., Hadjidj, A., Bouabdallah, A., & Challal, Y. (2016, February 01). Healing on the cloud: Secure cloud architecture for medical wireless sensor networks. *Future Generation Computer Systems, 55,* 266–277. https://doi.org/10.1016/j.future.2015.01.009

Matheny, M. E., Whicher, D., & Thadaney Israni, S. (2020, February 11). Artificial intelligence in health care: A report from the national academy of medicine. *JAMA, 323*(6), 509–510. https://doi.org/10.1001/jama.2019.21579

Mesko, B. (2019). *FDA approvals for smart algorithms in medicine in one giant infographic.* The Medical Futurist Institute. Retrieved 06/06/2019 from https://medicalfuturist.com/fda-approvals-for-algorithms-in-medicine/

Naik, N., Hameed, B. M. Z., Shetty, D. K., Swain, D., Shah, M., Paul, R., Aggarwal, K., Ibrahim, S., Patil, V., Smriti, K., Shetty, S., Rai, B. P., Chlosta, P., & Somani, B. K. (2022, March 14). Legal and ethical consideration in artificial intelligence in healthcare: Who takes responsibility? [Mini Review] *Frontiers in Surgery, 9.* https://doi.org/10.3389/fsurg.2022.862322

Nguyen, D. C., Pham, Q.-V., Pathirana, P. N., Ding, M., Seneviratne, A., Lin, Z., Dobre, O., & Hwang, W.-J. (2022). Federated learning for smart healthcare: A survey. *ACM Computing Surveys, 55*(3), Article 60. https://doi.org/10.1145/3501296

Obermeyer, Z., Powers, B., Vogeli, C., & Mullainathan, S. (2019, October 25). Dissecting racial bias in an algorithm used to manage the health of populations. *Science, 366*(6464), 447–453. https://doi.org/10.1126/science.aax2342

Ozaydin, B., Berner, E. S., & Cimino, J. J. (2021, January 01). Appropriate use of machine learning in healthcare. *Intelligence-Based Medicine, 5*, 100041. https://doi.org/10.1016/j.ibmed.2021.100041

Prosperi, M., Guo, Y., Sperrin, M., Koopman, J. S., Min, J. S., He, X., Rich, S., Wang, M., Buchan, I. E., & Bian, J. (2020, July 01). Causal inference and counterfactual prediction in machine learning for actionable healthcare. *Nature Machine Intelligence, 2*(7), 369–375. https://doi.org/10.1038/s42256-020-0197-y

Schwalbe, N., & Wahl, B. (2020, May 16). Artificial intelligence and the future of global health. *The Lancet, 395*(10236), 1579–1586. https://doi.org/10.1016/S0140-6736(20)30226-9

Shah, S. M., & Khan, R. A. (2020). Secondary use of electronic health record: Opportunities and challenges. *IEEE Access, 8*, 136947–136965. https://doi.org/10.1109/ACCESS.2020.3011099

Tong, C., Rocheteau, E., Veličković, P., Lane, N., & Liò, P. (2022). Predicting patient outcomes with graph representation learning. In A. Shaban-Nejad, M. Michalowski, & S. Bianco (Eds.), *AI for disease surveillance and pandemic intelligence: Intelligent disease detection in action* (pp. 281–293). Springer International Publishing. https://doi.org/10.1007/978-3-030-93080-6_20

Topol, E. J. (2019, January 01). High-performance medicine: The convergence of human and artificial intelligence. *Nature Medicine, 25*(1), 44–56. https://doi.org/10.1038/s41591-018-0300-7

Vishal, B. V., & Onkar, S. (2021). AI in healthcare market *Allied Market Research*. Retrieved 05/03/2023 from https://www.alliedmarketresearch.com/artificial-intelligence-in-healthcare-market

Wang, H., Wu, Q., Qin, B., & Domingo-Ferrer, J. (2014, August 01). FRR: Fair remote retrieval of outsourced private medical records in electronic health networks. *Journal of Biomedical Informatics, 50*, 226–233. https://doi.org/10.1016/j.jbi.2014.02.008

Wood, A., Najarian, K., & Kahrobaei, D. (2020). Homomorphic encryption for machine learning in medicine and bioinformatics. *ACM Computing Surveys, 53*(4), Article 70. https://doi.org/10.1145/3394658

Yang, J.-J., Li, J.-Q., & Niu, Y. (2015, February 01). A hybrid solution for privacy preserving medical data sharing in the cloud environment. *Future Generation Computer Systems, 43–44*, 74–86. https://doi.org/10.1016/j.future.2014.06.004

Further Reading

OECD. (n.d.). AI principles. Retrieved from https://oecd.ai/en/ai-principles

U.S. Department of Health & Human Services. (n.d.). HIPAA for individuals. Retrieved from https://www.hhs.gov/hipaa/for-individuals/index.html

5

Barriers and Solutions to Adoption of AI in Healthcare

Piyush Mathur

Cleveland Clinic, Cleveland, OH, USA

Bart Geerts

Healthplus.AI, Amsterdam, Netherlands

LEARNING OBJECTIVES

- Understand key barriers to the clinical adoption of AI in healthcare.
- Describe some solutions and frameworks that can facilitate trust and the adoption of AI in healthcare.
- Discuss how the demonstration of value proposition and improvement in the human–computer interface can accelerate clinician acceptance of AI in healthcare solutions.

Introduction

Healthcare is evolving by adopting and integrating various Artificial Intelligence (AI) systems into clinical and administrative practices. These systems are now available for clinician use for the majority of healthcare specialties, ranging from use in echocardiography amongst critically ill patients to determining the diagnosis of skin cancer in an outpatient setting. Such AI-enabled healthcare solutions have the potential to democratize care and provide greater access to healthcare providers as some of these solutions seek to be autonomous, such as that for diabetic retinopathy screening. The adoption of these AI solutions, as with the introduction of drugs or devices, will only advance when clinicians accept the algorithms' results and their applicability to their patient care. Despite years of continued growth in research related to AI in healthcare, there is still a significant gap in terms of the translation and clinical adoption of these systems (Toh, Dondelinger, & Wang, 2019). A lack of understanding, the reproducibility crisis, and issues relating to trust in the guidance provided by these algorithms, ineffective value proposition and a poor human–computer interface are among the challenges that are

DOI: 10.1201/9781003262152-5

cited as barriers to the clinical adoption of these algorithms (Stupple, Singerman, & Celi, 2019). In this chapter we describe the key factors representing barriers to the clinician adoption of rapidly developing AI solutions in healthcare and pragmatic approaches to overcoming them.

Clinician Education and Understanding of AI

While clinicians are increasingly excited to learn about AI and its possible use in their clinical practice, unfortunately there is a general lack of understanding of AI, and also how to evaluate it for appropriate clinical use. As AI solutions make their way to the bedside, clinicians, and not simply physicians, will need to be educated in the evaluation and use of these technologies (Keane & Topol, 2021). There has been a broader discussion on integrating AI education into the medical school curriculum. One particular study that examined the perceptions of future physicians on the possible influences of Artificial Intelligence on medicine and to determine the needs that might be helpful for curriculum restructuring involved some 3,018 medical students. Most of these participants perceived AI as an assistive technology that could facilitate physicians' access to information (85.8%) and patients to healthcare (76.7%) and also reduce errors (70.5%) (Civaner, Uncu, Bulut, Chalil, & Tatli, 2022). Of all the participants, only 6.0% stated that they were competent enough to inform patients about the features and risks of artificial intelligence. They further expressed their educational gaps regarding their need for "knowledge and skills related to artificial intelligence applications" (96.2%), "applications for reducing medical errors" (95.8%), and "training to prevent and solve ethical problems that might arise as a result of using artificial intelligence applications" (93.8%).

As a minimum, there is a defined need for clinicians to be able to read and understand AI studies. Faes et al. describe the key AI terms and methods and then provide a framework to evaluate an AI solution using a three-step process of deriving, validating, and establishing the clinical effectiveness of the tool (Faes et al., 2020). They describe how the type of AI model used, and its appropriateness for the input data type and data set size should be performed. Additionally, it is crucial to learn about the additional prespecified settings called hyperparameters, which must be tuned on a data set independent of the validation set (Liu, Chen, Krause, & Peng, 2019). On the validation set, the outcome against which the model is evaluated is termed the reference standard. Clinical evaluation for utility, considerations for clinical implementation and algorithm maintenance challenges have all been well addressed by Liu et al. Zhang et al. have even developed a framework to automate the assessment of mature publications in this era of ever-increasing publications related to AI in healthcare (Zhang et al., 2022). Using state-of-the-art Bi-directional Encoder Representations from Transformers Natural Language Processing (NLP) models with pre-training on medical corpora, their pipeline correctly classified 98% of the publications for inclusion and maturity when evaluated against publications discovered by recent systematic reviews. Such tools will prove very useful in screening publications which are rapidly expanding both quantitatively and qualitatively (Awasthi et al., 2023).

Another approach is to utilize less intense training methods, such as no coding learning, which have been rapidly gaining development and adoption. No-code learning can potentially expose learners to the critical principles of AI without the extensive requirement to build the code, which is a substantial barrier (Faes et al., 2019). Also, for continuous learning in an evolving field such as computer science, many of these coding languages and their associated solutions evolve rapidly. Most clinicians will not be expected to keep us with these changes. Hence, no-code models might be a better solution to keep their focus on the modelling and validation part. These can also be used to promote hands-on learning while doing cross-collaborative projects amongst clinicians and to lower the barriers to entry.

CASE STUDY 1   NO-CODE LEARNING FOR CLINICIAN EDUCATION (FAES ET AL., 2019)

INTRODUCTION

No-code development of machine learning models provides an opportunity to clinicians to introduce a lower barrier to learn key elements of AI model development and evaluation. This will mean that clinicians, in a more efficient manner, will be able to get hands-on training without the prerequisites to learn complex computer programming languages.

AI INTERVENTION

The researchers using Google CloudAutoML and data from five publicly available open-source datasets-built classification models to classify commonly occurring diseases.

RESULTS

Internal validations for the binary classification tasks using sensitivity specificity and Area under the Precision Recall Curve (AUPRC), achieved high value ranges of 73.3–97.0%, 67–100%, 0.87–1.00, respectively. However, the performance using the same parameters for the classification of multiple tasks, and in an external validation, was much lower.

KEY POINT

The authors concluded that the availability of automated deep learning platforms provides an opportunity for the medical community to enhance their understanding of the model development and evaluation.

Frameworks on evolving the medical education curriculum to include AI have also been proposed (Paranjape, Schinkel, Nannan Panday, Car, & Nanayakkara, 2019). These frameworks include the knowledge of mathematical concepts, AI fundamentals, data science, and related ethical and legal issues. These key skill sets might empower clinicians to understand the workings of AI tools, evaluate their accuracy, assess their applicability for appropriate case scenarios and even encourage the development of their innovative solutions. Such proposals have included considering making high-quality web-based courses on data sciences and AI fundamentals freely offered in the core phase of medical education. This might lead to students focusing on the applications of these subjects more naturally in the following years of training. Many of these courses are already available through massive open online courses (MOOCs) (Liyanagunawardena & Williams, 2014). In a graduated manner, these proposals recommend that for both residents and medical students who have already finished this phase of training, courses on the fundamental subjects should be available and mandatory throughout the remaining part of their medical education.

Similarly, introductory courses and refresher courses should also be made available for practicing physicians. It will be essential to start with a "train-the-trainer" approach in order that there is a sufficient number of trainers to guide the screening and development of appropriate courses and curricula. This core group would also be fundamentally important in working with AI domain experts to review changes to the ever-evolving science related to AI itself. Regulatory bodies such as ACGME might need to form specific task forces to guide and supervise, such as with regard to curriculum content. Similar frameworks will also be necessary for education amongst non-clinician healthcare providers, as many of these technologies will be used by them.

Trust, Reproducibility & Explainability

One essential aspect of the adoption of trust in the guidance being delivered by the AI algorithm. Trust has been described as a human belief that is broadly defined based on three main dimensions: benevolence, integrity, and ability. Part of this is from a foundational lack of understanding of these algorithms' functions. Still, there are other components, such as users' past experiences, user biases, and perception towards automation, as well as properties of the AI system, including controllability, transparency, and complexity of the model, associated risks, explainability, interpretability, reliability and reproducibility of the guidance that play an essential role (Figure 5.1). These components might be different for the patients from clinicians, who depend on guidance from clinicians for shared decision-making, emphasizing the role of trust in shared decision-making (Asan, Bayrak, & Choudhury, 2020).

Among these factors, reliability, which refers to whether the AI technology can perform a task predictably and consistently, might be particularly concerning in healthcare due to the changes in the reliability of AI in the presence of new data. Additionally, other limitations, including governance, reproducibility, and interpretation, have been outlined by Toh et al. (Toh et al., 2019). Aspects of the lack of understanding include the determination of the accuracy parameters and applicability of the algorithm for specific clinical scenarios. The generalizability of AI algorithms' results and their reproducibility amongst different health setups or patient populations has been very challenging. Part of these issues stem from the limitations of the datasets these algorithms have been trained on, and intrinsically they may carry biases, limiting their generalizability. But implementation also poses significant challenges as the data or model performance may differ.

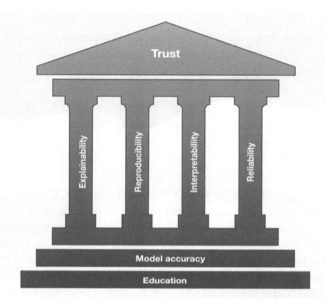

FIGURE 5.1
Foundational and supportive factors essential for clinician trust in AI system guidance.

(Source: Authors.)

CASE STUDY 2   CLINICIAN ADOPTING A HYPOTENSION PREDICTION ALGORITHM (MAHESHWARI ET AL., 2020)

INTRODUCTION

An algorithm (Hypotension Prediction Index, HPI), based on machine learning, was developed which predicts intraoperative hypotension within 15 minutes of its occurrence with a sensitivity, specificity and an area under the receiver operating characteristics (AUROC) of 88%, 87% and 0.95, respectively.

AI INTERVENTION

The algorithm performance was studies in the operating room. Its guidance alerted the clinicians to possible hypotension event when the index exceeded 85 (range, 0–100). In addition, it also provided recommendations on vasopressor administration, fluid administration, inotrope administration, or just observation.

RESULTS

Among the 214 patients who were enrolled for the study, guidance was provided for 105(49%) of the patients randomly assigned to the index group. The index guidance in these patients did not reduce the amount of hypotension in the guidance group compared to the unguided group ($p = 0.75$). In the post hoc analysis, the investigators found less hypotension when the clinicians intervened followed the guidance.

KEY POINT

The authors found that half of the guidance alerts were not followed by treatments due to various possibilities including short warning time, complex treatment, or clinicians ignoring the alert.

Celi et al. have suggested that data and code-sharing standards must transition from mere publication policies to allow third parties to reproduce studies (Celi, Citi, Ghassemi, & Pollard, 2019). They also recommended developing guidelines for reporting and evaluating results, such as those for causal inference and reinforcement learning studies, which must be refined and expanded across the field. Along the same lines, they described increasing fairness and transparency and ensuring robustness in developing these algorithms to improve trust (Asan et al., 2020). To address these gaps, especially during the translation from research to early implementation, guidelines such as Developmental and Exploratory Clinical Investigations of DEcision support systems driven by Artificial Intelligence (DECIDE-AI, provide a framework incorporating seventeen AI-specific reporting items and ten generic reporting items (Vasey et al., 2022). Similarly, the 'Translational Evaluation of Healthcare AI (TEHAI)' evaluation framework is designed to address these translational gaps along the three critical components of capability, utility and adoption at any stage of the development and deployment of the AI system (Reddy et al., 2021).

A survey of 400 algorithms presented at the two leading AI conferences shows that only 6% of the presenters have shared their implementation code, around 30% shared data, and only 50% shared "pseudocode" publicly (Gundersen, Gil, & Aha, 2018). Reproducibility has been described as one of the essential questions in AI research, in general, and not just limited to healthcare (Carter, Attia, Lopez-Jimenez, & Friedman, 2019). Carter et al. argue that there is a compelling need to find a way to share data and programs to ensure reproducibility while protecting patient privacy, financial investments, and intellectual property. Amongst the various solutions described by them, including sharing data and programming code, development of a shared protected computing environment, an appropriate license agreement, an application that houses the trained algorithm and necessary support code to run the algorithm, the mixed-media approach of combining written technical summaries in the form of a manuscript with runtime video capture showing the compilation and utilization of the computing environment is by far the most pragmatic.

More than the technical methods, interdisciplinary collaboration between AI researchers and clinicians is vital to the development of explainable models. In a review of explainable artificial intelligence (XAI) models that use real-world electronic health record data, the authors found more than 26% of the articles did not explicitly report any evaluation of the XAI method they used (Payrovnaziri et al., 2020). As outlined, some of the critical challenges leading to the lack of explainability in models were related to interpretable visualizations, the absence of a consistent definition, and the lack of clear evidence for uncommon diseases. They described solutions which could be grouped into five categories to address model explainability: 1) feature interaction and importance, 2) attention mechanism, 3) data dimensionality reduction, 4) knowledge distillation and rule extraction, and 5) intrinsically interpretable models (Payrovnaziri et al., 2020). Out of these methods, attention mechanism, feature interaction and importance (60%) were described as the top approaches.

Demonstrating Value Proposition

One of the significant barriers to the clinical adoption of AI in healthcare is the lack of clear demonstration of the value proposition. Healthcare organizations and providers hesitate to invest in and use AI technologies without relevant evidence. To overcome this barrier, AI-system manufacturers (which can also be the hospitals themselves, by the way) must demonstrate their solutions' value proposition through rigorous testing and evaluation.

The type of evidence that needs to be provided also varies for each solution, the different stakeholders, and the kind of healthcare system (i.e., national health insurance or out-of-pocket model). The various stakeholders, by and large, are the patient, the clinical specialist, the manager, the board member, an insurance company or other payor, and the regulatory authority.

An essential framework that can be used to include all stakeholders is, of course, the quadruple aim (Bodenheimer & Sinsky, 2014). But it all starts with AI developers working closely with clinicians and/or patients to identify specific pain points and challenges in clinical workflows and develop solutions that directly address these issues. The best framework to use to find the metrics to demonstrate value for different stakeholders will depend on the specific goals and objectives of the AI system in question, as well as the needs and priorities of the healthcare organization and its stakeholders.

The value proposition needs to be demonstrated in clinical trials and studies assessing AI algorithms' effectiveness and safety in real-world healthcare settings.

AI systems often come to market with limited proof of value, mere mathematical evidence of performance and robustness in test, internal and (sometimes) external validations. Consequently, multicenter trials are required to study the impact on clinical behavior, outcomes, and economic implications.

It is essential to point out that several methodologies currently go unused that can fill the gap of a lack of prospective clinical and economic research in the initial stages of the AI system that is introduced. The pre-clinical impact assessment, the net-benefit analysis and the (early) health technology assessment can be good and relatively low-cost tools to add certainty in the early validation stages (Vickers, Van Calster, & Steyerberg, 2016). In the end, we need clear prospective evidence of AI systems' clinical and economic benefits. In a review of AI technologies for the ICU, it becomes apparent that only 2% of solutions get prospectively and clinically validated; this needs to improve to remove providers' hesitations to invest in and use AI.

Finally, AI manufacturers need to be transparent about their solutions' (potential) limitations and risks and work closely with healthcare providers and regulators to address these concerns.

Usability & Feasibility: The Human–Computer Interface

The human–computer interface (HCI) refers to the interaction between the healthcare provider and the AI system. The success of the clinical adoption of AI in healthcare relies heavily on effective HCI, which presents a significant barrier in the current landscape. The increasing relevance and importance of HCI are stressed in the DECIDE-AI guideline (Vasey et al., 2021). And we see more and more manufacturers in healthcare work with user-centered design, UI (user interface), and UX (user experience) approaches.

Integration into the existing clinical workflows and systems is essential in ensuring that an AI system delivers its value. Procedures involve developing seamless interfaces and integrations with electronic health records (EHRs) and other clinical processes and providing training and support to ensure that healthcare providers are comfortable and proficient in using the technology. Here several challenges in the HCI become apparent:

- AI models may produce results that are difficult to interpret or understand by clinicians leading to mistrust and skepticism towards AI systems.
- A lack of standardization in AI systems: Different AI systems may use different user interfaces, which can be confusing and frustrating for clinicians navigating multiple systems.
- Integration of AI systems into clinical workflows can be challenging.
- The challenge mentioned above is to communicate limitations and provide explainable results concisely.

To address these challenges, HCI design should prioritize user-centered design that can be easily understood and navigated when designing AI systems.

Conclusion

Healthcare is evolving rapidly as it adopts various AI systems into its practices. The adoption of these AI solutions, like the adoption of drugs or devices, will only advance when clinicians accept the algorithms' results and their applicability to their patient care. The major barriers need to be overcome with some of the recommended solutions to foster clinical adoption of AI systems (Table 5.1).

TABLE 5.1

Barriers and Recommended Solutions for Clinician Adoption of AI Systems

Barrier	Solution
Education	• Integrated AI curriculum for medical trainees. • Educational programs and research funds for tiered clinician education.
Trust	• Research and development to address key components of trust in AI systems (e.g., Explainability). • Evaluation frameworks for assessment of AI systems(e.g., TEHAI framework).
Value proposition	• Business case methodology development. • Clinical and cost-effectiveness evaluation of AI systems.
Human–computer interface	• Human-centered design. • Early involvement of clinicians in AI system design.

SUMMARY

- There is still a significant gap between research and translation to the clinical practice of AI algorithms in healthcare.

- This gap has various reasons, including trust, the reproducibility of results, explainability, value proposition, clinician education and poor human–computer interfaces.

- Clinician education is lacking, and there is an opportunity to use available resources to bridge this gap.

- Challenges with the reproducibility of results delivered by these AI algorithms create an environment of mistrust.

- The value proposition needs to be demonstrated for cost-effective improvements in care delivery using these AI algorithms to facilitate clinician adoption.

- Human–computer interface design is essential to understanding and navigating AI systems integrated into clinician workflow.

REVIEW QUESTIONS

- Identify the critical barriers to the clinical adoption of AI algorithms.

- How can clinician trust be built in the guidance provided by the AI algorithms?

- What role does clinician education in AI play in improving understanding and adoption of AI-based clinical guidance?

- How can a value proposition be created to justify the adoption of AI algorithms providing clinical guidance?

- Do human–computer interfaces have a role in improving the usability and adoption of AI algorithm-based clinical guidance?

References

Asan, O., Bayrak, A. E., & Choudhury, A. (2020). Artificial intelligence and human trust in healthcare: Focus on clinicians. *J Med Internet Res*, 22(6), e15154. doi:10.2196/15154

Awasthi, R., Mishra, S., Cywinski, J. B., Maheshwari, K., Khanna, A. K., Papay, F. A., & Mathur, P. (2023). Quantitative and qualitative evaluation of the recent artificial intelligence in healthcare publications using deep-learning. *medRxiv*, 2022.2012.2031.22284092. doi:10.1101/2022.12.31.22284092

Bodenheimer, T., & Sinsky, C. (2014). From triple to quadruple aim: care of the patient requires care of the provider. *Ann Fam Med*, 12(6), 573–576. doi:10.1370/afm.1713

Carter, R. E., Attia, Z. I., Lopez-Jimenez, F., & Friedman, P. A. (2019). Pragmatic considerations for fostering reproducible research in artificial intelligence. *NPJ Digit Med*, 2, 42. doi:10.1038/s41746-019-0120-2

Celi, L. A., Citi, L., Ghassemi, M., & Pollard, T. J. (2019). The PLOS ONE collection on machine learning in health and biomedicine: Towards open code and open data. *PLoS One*, 14(1), e0210232. doi:10.1371/journal.pone.0210232

Civaner, M. M., Uncu, Y., Bulut, F., Chalil, E. G., & Tatli, A. (2022). Artificial intelligence in medical education: A cross-sectional needs assessment. *BMC Med Educ*, 22(1), 772. doi:10.1186/s12909-022-03852-3

Faes, L., Liu, X., Wagner, S. K., Fu, D. J., Balaskas, K., Sim, D. A., … Denniston, A. K. (2020). A clinician's guide to artificial intelligence: How to critically appraise machine learning studies. *Transl Vis Sci Technol*, 9(2), 7. doi:10.1167/tvst.9.2.7

Faes, L., Wagner, S. K., Fu, D. J., Liu, X., Korot, E., Ledsam, J. R., … Keane, P. A. (2019). Automated deep learning design for medical image classification by health-care professionals with no coding experience: A feasibility study. *Lancet Digit Health*, 1(5), e232–e242. doi:10.1016/S2589-7500(19)30108-6

Gundersen, O. E., Gil, Y., & Aha, D. W. (2018). On reproducible AI: Towards reproducible research, open science, and digital scholarship in AI publications. *AI Magazine*, 39(3), 56–68. doi:10.1609/aimag.v39i3.2816

Keane, P. A., & Topol, E. J. (2021). AI-facilitated health care requires education of clinicians. *Lancet*, 397(10281), 1254. doi:10.1016/S0140-6736(21)00722-4

Liu, Y., Chen, P. C., Krause, J., & Peng, L. (2019). How to read articles that use machine learning: Users' guides to the medical literature. *JAMA*, 322(18), 1806–1816. doi:10.1001/jama.2019.16489

Liyanagunawardena, T. R., & Williams, S. A. (2014). Massive open online courses on health and medicine: Review. *J Med Internet Res*, 16(8), e191. doi:10.2196/jmir.3439

Maheshwari, K., Shimada, T., Yang, D., Khanna, S., Cywinski, J. B., Irefin, S. A., … Sessler, D. I. (2020). Hypotension prediction index for prevention of hypotension during moderate- to high-risk noncardiac surgery. *Anesthesiology*, 133(6), 1214–1222. doi:10.1097/ALN.0000000000003557

Paranjape, K., Schinkel, M., Nannan Panday, R., Car, J., & Nanayakkara, P. (2019). Introducing artificial intelligence training in medical education. *JMIR Med Educ*, 5(2), e16048. doi:10.2196/16048

Payrovnaziri, S. N., Chen, Z., Rengifo-Moreno, P., Miller, T., Bian, J., Chen, J. H., … He, Z. (2020). Explainable artificial intelligence models using real-world electronic health record data: A systematic scoping review. *J Am Med Inform Assoc*, 27(7), 1173–1185. doi:10.1093/jamia/ocaa053

Reddy, S., Rogers, W., Makinen, V. P., Coiera, E., Brown, P., Wenzel, M., … Kelly, B. (2021). Evaluation framework to guide implementation of AI systems into healthcare settings. *BMJ Health Care Inform*, 28(1). doi:10.1136/bmjhci-2021-100444

Stupple, A., Singerman, D., & Celi, L. A. (2019). The reproducibility crisis in the age of digital medicine. *NPJ Digit Med*, 2, 2. doi:10.1038/s41746-019-0079-z

Toh, T. S., Dondelinger, F., & Wang, D. (2019). Looking beyond the hype: Applied AI and machine learning in translational medicine. *EBioMedicine*, *47*, 607–615. doi:10.1016/j.ebiom.2019.08.027

Vasey, B., Clifton, D. A., Collins, G. S., Denniston, A. K., Faes, L., Geerts, B. F., … The, D.-A. I. S. G. (2021). DECIDE-AI: New reporting guidelines to bridge the development-to-implementation gap in clinical artificial intelligence. *Nature Medicine*, *27*(2), 186–187. doi:10.1038/s41591-021-01229-5

Vasey, B., Nagendran, M., Campbell, B., Clifton, D. A., Collins, G. S., Denaxas, S., … McCulloch, P. (2022). Reporting guideline for the early stage clinical evaluation of decision support systems driven by artificial intelligence: DECIDE-AI. *BMJ*, *377*, e070904. doi:10.1136/bmj-2022-070904

Vickers, A. J., Van Calster, B., & Steyerberg, E. W. (2016). Net benefit approaches to the evaluation of prediction models, molecular markers, and diagnostic tests. *BMJ*, *352*, i6. doi:10.1136/bmj.i6

Zhang, J., Whebell, S., Gallifant, J., Budhdeo, S., Mattie, H., Lertvittayakumjorn, P., … Teo, J. T. (2022). An interactive dashboard to track themes, development maturity, and global equity in clinical artificial intelligence research. *Lancet Digit Health*, *4*(4), e212–e213. doi:10.1016/S2589-7500(22)00032-2

6

Ethics, Regulation and Legal Issues of AI in Healthcare

Sandra Johnson

University of Sydney School of Medicine, Sydney, Australia

Sandeep Reddy

Deakin School of Medicine, Geelong, Australia

LEARNING OBJECTIVES

- Recognising the importance of regulation and ethics in AI
- Understanding bias in data
- Learn the principal factors in the regulation of data
- Note the importance of ongoing monitoring and vigilance when AI systems are implemented

Introduction

Artificial Intelligence (AI) has become increasingly integrated into our daily lives, from the use of virtual assistants like Siri and Alexa to self-driving cars and medical diagnosis systems. However, the development and deployment of AI raises numerous ethical concerns. At this time in our history, we have the capacity to influence the future through ethical application and interaction with AI so that we can arrive at a human–AI inter-relationship that leads to greater well-being for humankind. Without the adoption of an ethical approach to regulation and governance, there is the risk that highly intelligent systems could be left unmonitored, or, at worst, be placed in the hands of those driven by self-interest and power. This chapter will explore the ethical considerations related to AI and provide an overview of some of the ethical and regulatory frameworks that can be used to guide the development and use of AI.

AI is discussed in some detail in the previous chapters of this book. For the purposes of this chapter AI is defined as the study of intelligent devices or agents that can perceive their surroundings and take appropriate action to maximize the chance of achieving an objective (Rong, Mendez et al., 2020). Another interesting definition, offered by the

DOI: 10.1201/9781003262152-6

mathematician, Dobrev (2012), is that "AI will be such a program which in an arbitrary world will cope no worse than a human."

Ethics of AI in Healthcare

Physicians are aware of the importance of ethics in patient management, as emphasized in Beauchamp and Childress' *Principles of Biomedical Ethics* (1994). The principles that are applied in clinical practice and in scientific research are primarily autonomy, beneficence, non-maleficence, and justice. They include primarily respect for the patient's right to make independent decisions about their medical treatment (autonomy); the treatment aim is to benefit the patient (beneficence); the treating doctor must at all times act in the patient's best interest to ensure that no harm occurs to the patient (non-maleficence) and the doctor must ensure that fairness and equity in access to services is applied in the management of the patient's condition (justice). Whilst these are ethical principles, there are also significant legal implications for doctors where respect for patient autonomy and informed consent is paramount in patient care.

We cannot assume that the same ethical principles are applied when technology designers and digital scientists manufacture devices for healthcare. Many ethical guidelines have been released in recent years in disciplines such as engineering, medicine, data science and law. Business relies on income from sales and in such a setting ethics could be a low priority. Often business supports science in the development of new technologies that may impact on individuals in society and in some instances AI experiments are done on members of society without informed consent (Kramer et al., 2014). Privacy invasion by social media Apps is another example of such activity. The whistle-blower Frances Haugen spoke out about the inherent problem associated with the lack of regulation of Facebook as a holder of personal information in their social media Apps (Persily, 2021). This example is given merely to illustrate that regulation is needed when individual's data is used for purposes beyond that for which it was intended. Another recent example from Australia occurred when a telecommunications company, Optus, was hacked and information such as passport details, driver's licence, birth dates, phone numbers, healthcare information and addresses were hacked from the system. Essentially, Optus retained details of individuals beyond the initial purpose of identification when the accounts were opened. The Australian Government is now considering stricter regulation about companies retaining personal data. It is essential that such regulation and governance occurs in many areas where individuals interact with online systems.

In AI device and program development, academics can be funded by private companies and in this relationship a valid question is: who controls the data and who is responsible for the privacy of that data? One could argue that companies that receive funding from manufacturers and designers are at risk of bias when it comes to ethical considerations in the development of products. It is important that we do not stifle innovation, but we should expect open disclosure about the true intent of the device or App when it is likely to influence or impact on the well-being of members of society. We live in a world where we are more connected than ever before in our history. The concept of Web Intelligence, which is considered to be an enhancement of AI and IT, is growing where multidisciplinary research in areas like data science, human-centred computing and network services is increasing (Kuai et al., 2022) (Zhong, et al., 2000).

The development of human-centric AI will require the collaboration of multidisciplinary experts in data science, machine learning, software designers, social psychologists, ethics, healthcare and law as well as the public to ensure that critical factors such as privacy, data ownership, accountability, transparency and fairness are respected. Technical solutions to these issues are suggested in an article by Lepri et al. (2021).

> ### CASE STUDY 1   RACIAL BIAS IN AN ALGORITHM USED TO MANAGE THE HEALTH OF POPULATIONS (OBERMEYER ET AL., 2019)
>
> Obermeyer et al. (2019) found that one algorithm used by Optum, a subsidiary of UnitedHealth Group, had been discriminating against black patients in the US healthcare system. The algorithm was designed to identify high-risk patients to allocate funds in the healthcare system based on healthcare costs. However, due to the historic racial disparities in access to care, the algorithm had a racial bias, resulting in only 17.7% of black patients being identified as high-risk, while the true number should have been 46.5%. The algorithm's bias presented not only a discrimination problem but also harm to individual patients by hindering physicians from intervening in advance of a medical crisis.
>
> The racial bias in Optum's algorithm is, by far, the only publicly available evidence of discrimination resulting from biases in AI in the healthcare context. While discrimination as a result of biases in AI is well documented in other fields, this study highlights the importance of addressing ethical concerns related to the use of AI in healthcare and the potential for biased algorithms to lead to unequal healthcare outcomes for different groups of people.

Ethical Frameworks

One of the primary ethical concerns related to AI is bias. Machine learning algorithms are only as unbiased as the data used to train them, and if the data is biased, the algorithm will be biased. This can result in the unfair treatment of individuals or groups and perpetuate systemic discrimination. For example, facial recognition technology has been shown to be less accurate in identifying people with darker skin tones, leading to potential misidentification and harm. Another concern is the potential impact of AI on employment. As AI and automation become more prevalent, there is a risk of significant job loss, particularly in industries like manufacturing and transportation. This could lead to economic inequality and social unrest. AI also raises concerns about privacy and data protection. With the vast amount of data collected by AI systems, there is a risk of misuse or abuse of personal information. Additionally, there is a potential for AI systems to be used for surveillance purposes, which could have significant implications for civil liberties. Finally, there are concerns about the accountability and transparency of AI systems. It can be difficult to determine how decisions are made by complex AI algorithms, making it challenging to assign responsibility in cases of harm or error. This lack of transparency can also lead to a lack of trust in AI systems.

Several ethical frameworks can be used to guide the development and use of AI. One commonly cited framework consists of the principles of transparency, fairness, and accountability (TFA). This framework emphasizes the need for transparency in AI decision-making processes, fairness in the treatment of individuals, and accountability for the outcomes of AI systems. Another framework is the Asilomar AI Principles, developed by a group of AI researchers and industry leaders in 2017. These principles include a commitment to safety, transparency, and alignment with human values. They also call for caution in the development and deployment of AI and emphasize the importance of considering the potential risks and benefits.

A third framework is the IEEE Global Initiative on Ethics of Autonomous and Intelligent Systems (n.d.), which provides a comprehensive set of guidelines for ethical AI development and deployment. These guidelines include a focus on transparency, accountability, and the protection of privacy and data.

Regulation of AI in Healthcare

Regulation occurs when a set of rules is applied by a government or an authority with the aim of controlling the behaviour of people or the way an activity is performed. A benchmark is set with standards or guidelines that need to be followed by the entities involved in the regulated behaviour. Whilst guidelines provide a framework for action and implementation of AI devices and AI in healthcare, we recognise that guidelines alone do not carry the legal gravitas to ensure that they are adhered to. This is where governance and regulation will play an important role. In some instances, the internal ethical guidelines by large corporations could merely be aimed at placating the regulators and society to avoid criticism and scrutiny (Hagendorff, 2020). Failure to comply with guidelines, resulting in the loss of reputation and/or restriction on professional membership alone, does not necessarily lead to adherence to guidelines, where the intent is to keep patients and the community safe. There needs to be a legal framework within which the guidelines are applied so that there are significant consequences to practice when new AI systems are developed and employed without strict compliance.

With regulation, many factors need to be considered and these also fall into the realm of ethics and law in relation to AI in healthcare. The main factors in relation to regulation, ethics and law are considered here under specific headings but overlap occurs within all these factors:

a) Data privacy and security
b) Trustworthiness of the technology
c) Reliability of the technology

d) Fairness

e) Accountability

f) Vigilance and monitoring

a) *Data privacy and security*

Patient health and personal information requires a high level of privacy as very delicate information, which is only known to the treating doctor, is often shared in clinical practice. Traditionally, information shared between doctor and patient is strictly confidential and guarded with great care. With health information now held online, sensitive and personal information can be placed online that could be used against the individual if such information is not protected.

Applications on smartphones that monitor health and fitness need to be safeguarded against breach. In addition, control for the sharing of data should remain in the hands of the individual, with some understanding on their part that they are sharing their personal health records. The My Health Records Act 2012 (n.d.) refers to establishing a voluntary national public health system that aims to overcome the fragmentation of health information, to improve the availability and quality of health information, to reduce the occurrence of adverse medical events and the duplication of treatment and to improve the coordination and quality of healthcare offered by different healthcare providers (Australian Government, 2012).

The Privacy Act 1988 is legislation that covers the collection, use, storage and disclosure of personal information in both the federal public and the private sectors. The privacy principles covered in this legislation aims to protect all information about individuals and applies to personal data collection for any purpose. The law needs to remain agile in the face of rapidly evolving technology, but the important point here is that laws already exist to protect personal information.

b) *Trustworthiness of technology*

For us to trust AI, the information around a device or technology needs to be transparent regarding its purpose, its process and its limitations. For the clinician, it is imperative that the device does not cause unintended harm to the patient.

Essential in the process of trustworthiness is transparency. For the AI device to be transparent its processing and pathway to prediction or action needs to be explainable and interpretable.

Explainability is where the intrinsic details of a device can be explained to the user and interpretability is the ability of the device to provide a predictable action in a manner that the user can understand. Clearly, these characteristics are important in medicine and healthcare where AI devices are used in direct patient care. The doctor needs to understand what the device will do and needs to trust that the device is true to what it claims to do (European Commission, 2019). In addition, the device needs to be transparent about its limitations, so that steps can be taken to avert harm to humans, something which is important in-patient care for example. The EU's policy document (2019) on trustworthiness refers to characteristics such as human oversight, technical robustness, privacy and data governance, transparency, fairness, well-being and accountability and it is worthwhile being familiar with this document when regulation is being considered.

c) *Reliability*

Reliability of the device is based on the reliability of the data used to train the models in the development of the device. The level of reliability needs to be clear to the user, namely the clinician. The clinician needs to know that the device is doing what it claims to do and that it does so with the best possible accuracy and validity. Validity in this case is where the device has been trained on subject cases that are relevant to the clinical setting. If a device claims to be generalizable it might not be specific enough to the clinical situation where it is implemented, and the clinician needs to have a clear understanding of any misfit.

Reliability also relates to bias, whether human bias or machine bias, and the user needs to remain aware of hidden or historical bias. Human bias can occur at the data collection and insertion point where the gender, race and ethnicity are given precedence when they may not be strong factors in a particular study. Also, factors could be given importance at data insertion when they may not be as relevant as the researcher believes. That is, the personal bias of the researcher could influence the data at collection and insertion. These issues may be more likely in historic data where vigilance regarding bias might not have occurred (Stanford, 2020).

Machine bias could occur when an algorithm scales up minor differences in study cases in a manner that is unintended by the researchers. One example of this is found in the ethnic or racial bias occurred in the COMPASS Recidivism Algorithm tool, which was used to assess the risk of recidivism in a criminal setting. Analysis of the tool revealed that it was more likely to label black men as repeat offenders than white men (Angwin et al., 2016). This issue clearly relates not only to reliability but also to justice and fairness as one of the principles of ethics.

d) *Fairness*

Where an AI algorithm processes data and can impact on the lives of people it is important that the system is fair. Any discrimination based on sex, race, ethnicity or other needs to be avoided. Lepri et al. (2021) discuss the issue of algorithm fairness, in which statistical methods can be used to reduce inequities when groups are studied.

Fairness also relates to the minimization of bias, which is discussed above. An additional point to make is that we recognise historical bias in data which can be perpetuated over time. Once again, clinicians need to be aware when such potential bias is embedded in the data used to train an AI system that will be used in healthcare. We are in the early stages of work being done to eliminate bias from AI systems that are used in healthcare (Hobson & Ross, 2021).

e) *Accountability*

In terms of accountability, doctors have a duty of care to their patients which ensures that they get informed consent for treatment (Dwyer, 1998). When new AI devices or systems are used in patient diagnosis and treatment the patient needs to be informed. If a device has the potential to unintentionally harm the patient, consent is paramount. AI devices or systems should be regarded as tools to assist the doctor and therefore the doctor carries responsibility when such devices are used in patient care. If the device is faulty as per the manufacturer's design or production, then a shared responsibility with the manufacturer or designer is needed when harm is evident, and liability is considered. Wherever possible, the doctor should endeavour to ensure the reliability and safety of the device before it is used in patient care and management.

Accountability is linked to transparency. As mentioned, where data is used to develop a system, it needs to be clear how the data was gathered, whether or not it was fit for purpose and is the processing of the data in designing the device/system was reliable and trustworthy. In some circumstances, manufacturers could intentionally design an opaque system to protect their intellectual rights and this needs consideration in terms of the regulation and governance of AI systems (Barocas & Selbst, 2016).

f) *Vigilance and Monitoring*

Once AI systems are in regular use there is a risk that we could become complacent and reduce vigilance and monitoring of the systems. Automation bias where clinicians come to expect that the prediction from the AI system is correct without applying their clinical judgement to ensure that such is the case (Kathleen et al, 1996). Ultimately, clinicians must retain their clinical skills and judgement in patient management because the doctor has a "duty of care" to the patient and the patient has a trusted relationship with the doctor. In this privileged role the doctor must ensure that any application, whether AI or not, is safe for use in direct patient care. If there is any doubt about the system or device, then the shortcomings need to be explained to the patient and informed consent must be obtained.

AI systems that are in use over a period require re-evaluation and review because data drift and concept drift can occur over time, meaning that the processing of the data could become unpredictable, irrelevant and unreliable. Data drift is where changes in the properties of independent variables occur within an algorithm over time. Concept drift is where two data sets were originally created for one purpose, and they become increasingly inaccurate and irrelevant to each other over time (Patel, 2022).

Regulatory Frameworks

There are several key regulatory frameworks for AI in healthcare from around the world, as summarized in Table 6.1.

TABLE 6.1

List of Regulatory Frameworks from Across the World

Regulatory Framework	Description
European Union's General Data Protection Regulation (GDPR)	Regulates personal data use in AI systems, ensuring transparency, security, and individual rights protection.
United States Food and Drug Administration's (FDA) Pre-Market Approval (PMA) process	Ensures safety and effectiveness of medical devices and AI systems before their sale or use in the US.
World Health Organization (WHO) Global Strategy on Digital Health	Provides guidance on the development and use of digital health technologies, including AI, for improved health outcomes globally.
Medical Device Regulation (MDR) and In-Vitro Diagnostic Regulation (IVDR)	Regulations in the EU ensuring safety and performance of medical devices and AI systems used in healthcare.
Health Insurance Portability and Accountability Act (HIPAA)	US federal law ensuring the privacy and security of patient health information, including data collected and processed by AI systems.
Canadian Institutes of Health Research (CIHR) Ethical Framework for AI in Healthcare	Provides guidance on the ethical use of AI in healthcare, including issues related to patient privacy, consent, and bias.

Governance Frameworks

Artificial Intelligence (AI) is increasingly being used in healthcare, with the potential to improve patient care and outcomes. However, the use of AI in healthcare also raises a number of ethical, regulatory, safety, and quality concerns. As discussed above, in medicine it is the doctor's responsibility to be familiar with the design and intent for the use of devices before implementing in medical practice. The doctor must obtain informed consent from the patient before using the device or methodology in direct patient care. Whilst some may disagree because they believe that the manufacturer/designer should take some responsibility, it is the author's opinion that doctors have a legal duty of care to their patients and as such must ensure that when new devices or AI technologies are utilized in patient care that informed consent is obtained (Johnson, 2019). The safety and privacy protection for patients must remain at the forefront of consideration.

An AI system/device is essentially a tool in the doctor's kit and therefore the doctor should understand the capability of the system, its reliability and validity in the specific clinical situation. Whist an AI system or clinical decision system might be able to process data faster than a human, there are factors in clinical practice that require slow processing so that decisions are made with the patient in mind, their pathology and also their emotional vulnerability with respect to their disease or clinical presentation. At the current time, AI systems process the data in logical steps and AI does not have the ability to make abstractions or to consider the various emotional responses of the patient with respect to their illness. Humans need human contact when it comes to dealing with complex issues about understanding and dealing with their disease.

To address these concerns, the authors of this article propose a Governance Model for AI in Healthcare (GMAIH). The GMAIH comprises four main components: fairness, transparency, trustworthiness, and accountability. GMAIH addresses ethical, regulatory, safety, and quality concerns. The GMAIH comprises four main components: fairness, transparency, trustworthiness, and accountability. The model proposes that data governance panels be established to review training datasets for AI models to ensure data representation, and sufficiency. The authors suggest that normative standards for AI applications in healthcare should conform to biomedical ethical principles, particularly fairness, and should not lead to discrimination, disparity, or health inequities. The authors also recommend that explainable AI (XAI) be employed to enhance transparency, and that AI agents support patients' autonomy by providing transparent understanding sufficient to meet their individual requirements for decision-making. Lastly, the model proposes an emphasis on ongoing or continual explainability through interpretable frameworks, particularly for AI models that have explainability issues. The model also highlights the importance of trustworthiness, and the need for clinicians to understand the methods and models employed by AI applications.

The GMAIH is a comprehensive and well-considered framework for the responsible development and use of AI in healthcare. It addresses several key ethical, regulatory, safety, and quality concerns.

Other key governance frameworks for AI application in healthcare include:

1. "Ethical Guidelines for Trustworthy AI" by the European Commission's High-Level Expert Group on AI (2019). This framework provides a set of guidelines for the development and deployment of AI that is ethical, transparent, and respects human rights. It includes principles such as ensuring accountability, avoiding bias, and promoting transparency.

2. "Ethics and Governance of AI for Health" by the World Health Organization (2021). This report provides guidance on how to ensure that AI in healthcare is developed and used in an ethical and responsible way. It covers topics such as data governance, transparency, and accountability.

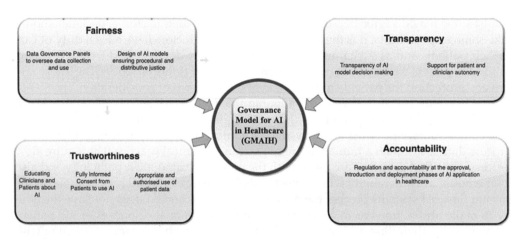

FIGURE 6.1
Governance model for AI in healthcare.

(Source: Reddy et al., 2020.)

3. "Ethics of Artificial Intelligence in Radiology" (Geis et al. 2019). This report provides a set of guidelines for the ethical and safe use of AI in radiology. It includes recommendations for data privacy, quality assurance, and transparency.

4. "The AI Ethics Impact Assessment Framework" by the Fujitsu (2022). This framework provides a step-by-step process for assessing the ethical implications of AI systems. It includes a set of questions to guide developers, policy-makers, and other stakeholders in identifying and addressing potential ethical concerns.

Conclusion

The emergence of global initiatives for experts who work in the field of AI represents a significant step forward in the responsible development and governance of AI technologies. These initiatives aim to bring together professionals from diverse backgrounds, including computer science, ethics, law, and social sciences, to address the complex challenges associated with AI. By collaborating and learning from one another, these experts can work towards ensuring that AI is developed and implemented in a way that benefits society, while minimizing the risks and negative consequences that may arise.

The field of AI is continuously evolving, and the challenges and ethical considerations associated with it are constantly changing. Therefore, it is essential that experts remain informed about the latest developments and best practices, and that they collaborate with colleagues from various disciplines to ensure the best possible outcomes for humans into the future. In this way, the responsible development and governance of AI can be seen as a shared responsibility, not only among experts but also among policy makers, industry leaders, and the wider public. Ultimately, it is through collaboration and ongoing learning that we can ensure that AI technologies are developed and implemented in a way that maximizes their potential benefits while minimizing their potential risks (Johnson, 2022).

SUMMARY

- AI is increasingly being used in healthcare
- Understanding bias in data and the potential for errors in algorithms
- The principles of privacy, trustworthiness, reliability, fairness, accountability, vigilance and monitoring are essential in the regulation process
- The doctor must always act in the best interest of patients when using AI technology and needs to understand the AI system being used
- Governance of AI is a shared responsibility across many sectors including healthcare and the broader community

REVIEW QUESTIONS

- What are some potential benefits of AI in healthcare?
- What are some ethical considerations that must be taken into account when implementing AI in healthcare?
- How can bias impact AI in healthcare?
- What are some legal concerns around AI in healthcare, particularly in relation to patient data?
- How does the current regulation of AI in healthcare compare to other industries?
- How can effective regulation of AI in healthcare be achieved?
- What role does innovation play in the regulation of AI in healthcare?
- What are some potential risks associated with using AI in healthcare?

References

AI HLEG. (2019). Ethics guidelines for trustworthy AI. *European Commission*. https://ec.europa.eu/newsroom/dae/document.cfm?doc_id=60419

Angwin, J., Larson, J., Mattu, S., & Kirchner, L. (2016). Machine bias. *ProPublica* https://www.propublica.org/article/machine-bias-risk-assessments-in-criminal-sentencing

Asilomar AI Principles. (2017). Future of Life Institute. https://futureoflife.org/ai-principles/

Australian Government. (2021). My Health Records Act 2012 - C2021C00475. Federal Register of Legislation. Retrieved from https://www.legislation.gov.au/Details/C2021C00475

Barocas, S., & Selbst, A. (2016). Big data's disparate impact. *California Law Review*, 104, 671–732.

Beauchamp, T., & Childress, J. (1994). *Principles of biomedical ethics* (4th ed.). Oxford University Press.

Bostrom, N., & Yudkowsky, E. (2020). Ethics of artificial intelligence and robotics. In E. N. Zalta (Ed.), *The Stanford encyclopedia of philosophy* (Spring 2020 Edition). https://plato.stanford.edu/archives/spr2020/entries/ethics-ai/

Dobrev, D. (2012). A definition of artificial intelligence. *arXiv preprint arXiv:1210.1568*.

Dwyer, P. (1998). Legal implications of clinical practice guidelines. *The Medical Journal of Australia*, 169(6), 292–293. https://doi.org/10.5694/j.1326-5377.1998.tb140275.x

Fujitsu. (2022). AI Ethics Whitepaper. Retrieved from https://www.fujitsu.com/global/documents/about/research/technology/aiethics/fujitsu-AIethics-whitepaper_en.pdf

Geis, J. R., Brady, A. P., Wu, C. C., Spencer, J., Ranschaert, E., Jaremko, J. L., Langer, S. G., Borondy Kitts, A., Birch, J., Shields, W. F., van den Hoven van Genderen, R., Kotter, E., Wawira Gichoya, J., Cook, T. S., Morgan, M. B., Tang, A., Safdar, N. M., & Kohli, M. (2019). Ethics of artificial intelligence in radiology: Summary of the joint European and North American multisociety statement. *Radiology*, 293(2), 436–440.

Hagendorff, T. (2020). The ethics of AI ethics: An evaluation of guidelines. *Minds and Machines*, 30, 99–120. https://doi.org/10.1007/s11023-020-09517-8

Hobson, C., & Ross, K. (2021). Removing data bias from AI and machine learning tools in health-care. *HIMSS*. https://www.himss.org/resources/removing-data-bias-ai-and-machine-learning-tools-healthcare-white-paper?utm_campaign=general&utm_source=google&utm_medium=cpc&utm_term=_&adgroupid=134509372449 &gclid=Cj0KCQjwn4qWBhCv ARIsAFNAMihhVZgMmvs4jWa7xomRDKvC3SAWljbFOOlE8EP9pUa4xRrh1w5PS 1IaAm1KEALw_wcB

IEEE Global Initiative on Ethics of Autonomous and Intelligent Systems. (n.d.). IEEE Standards Association. https://standards.ieee.org/industry-connections/ec/autonomous-systems.html

Jobin, A., Ienca, M., & Vayena, E. (2019). The global landscape of AI ethics guidelines. *Nature Machine Intelligence*, 1(9), 389–399. https://doi.org/10.1038/s42256-019-0088-2

Johnson, S. L. J. (2019). AI, machine learning, and ethics in health care. *Journal of Legal Medicine*, 39(4), 427–441. https://doi.org/10.1080/01947648.2019.1690604

Johnson, S. L. J. (2022). Artificial intelligence in health care: The challenge of effective regulation. *Journal of Legal Medicine*, 42(1–2), 75–86. https://doi.org/10.1080/01947648.2022.2158682

Kathleen, L. Mosier & Skitla, Linda J. (1996). Human decision makers and automated decision aids: Made for each other. In R. Parasuraman & M. Mouloua (Eds.), *Automation and human-performance: Theory and applications* (pp. 201–220).

Kramer, A. D. I., Guillory, J. E., & Hancock, J. T. (2014). Experimental evidence of massive-scale emotional contagion through social networks. *Proceedings of the National Academy of Sciences of the United States of America*, 111(24), 8788–8790.

Kuai, H., Tao, X., & Zhong, N. (2022). Web intelligence meets brain informatics: Towards the future of artificial intelligence in the connected world. *World Wide Web*, 25(4), 1223–1241. https://doi.org/10.1007/s11280-022-01030-5

Lepri, B., Oliver, N., & Pentland, A. (2021). Ethical machines: The human-centric use of artificial intelligence. *iScience*, 24, 102249. https://doi.org/10.1016/j.isci.2021.102249

Lipton, Z.C. (2016). The mythos of model interpretability. *Queue*, 16, 31–57.

Mosier, K. L., & Skitla, L. J. (1996). Human decision makers and automated decision aids: Made for each other. In R. Parasuraman & M. Mouloua (Eds)., *Automation and human performance*, 1st edition, CRC Press.

My Health Records Act 2012. (n.d.). https://www.legislation.gov.au/Details/C2019C00337

Obermeyer, Z., Powers, B., Vogeli, C., & Mullainathan, S. (2019). Dissecting racial bias in an algorithm used to manage the health of populations. *Science*, 336, 447.

Patel, H. (2022). Data drift and concept drift. https://harshilp.medium.com/what-is-concept-drift-and-why-does-it-go-undetected-9a84971565c0

Persily, N. (2021, October 5). What Congress needs to learn from Facebook whistleblower Frances Haugen. *The Washington Post*. https://www.washingtonpost.com/opinions/2021/10/05/what-congress-needs-learn-facebook-whistleblower-frances-haugen/

Reddy, S., Allan, S., Coghlan, S., & Cooper, P. (2020). A governance model for the application of AI in health care. *Journal of the American Medical Informatics Association*, 27(3), 491–497. https://doi.org/10.1093/jamia/ocz192

Review of My Health Records Legislation. (2020). https://www.health.gov.au/resources/collections/review-of-the-my-health-records-legislation

Rong, G., Mendez, A., et al. (2020). Artificial intelligence in healthcare: Review and prediction case studies. *Journal of Pre-proofs*, 6(3), 291–301.

Takshi, S. (2021). Unexpected inequality: Disparate-impact from artificial intelligence in health-care decisions. *Journal of Law and Health*, 34, 215.

World Health Organization (2021). *Ethics and governance of artificial intelligence for health: WHO guidance*. Geneva: World Health Organization.

Zhong, N., Liu, J., Yao, Y., & Ohsuga, S. (2000). Web intelligence (WI). In *Proceedings 24th Annual International Computer Software and Applications Conference. COMPSAC2000*, pp. 469–470. IEEE Computer Society.

Further Reading

Johnson, S. L. J. (2022). Artificial intelligence in health care: The challenge of effective regulation. *Journal of Legal Medicine*, 42(1–2), 75–86. https://doi.org/10.1080/01947648.2022.2158682

Reddy, S., Allan, S., Coghlan, S., & Cooper, P. (2020). A governance model for the application of AI in health care. *Journal of the American Medical Informatics Association: JAMIA*, 27(3), 491–497.

7

Translational Challenges of Implementing AI in Healthcare: Solutions and Opportunities

Dwarikanath Mahapatra

Inception AI, Abu Dhabi, UAE

Sandeep Reddy

Deakin School of Medicine, Geelong, Australia

LEARNING OBJECTIVES

- Describe the different technical challenges in implementing AI in healthcare.
- Identify the potential solutions for addressing these challenges.
- Explain why establishing trust is important in implementing AI in healthcare.
- Assess the potential risks and benefits of implementing AI in healthcare.

Introduction

Artificial Intelligence (AI) has the potential to revolutionize the healthcare industry by providing new opportunities for improving patient outcomes and reducing costs. However, some misconceptions suggest that AI in healthcare means simply replacing physicians with machines, which is emphatically not the case. In fact, the scope of AI in healthcare is broad and complex. It can encompass a wide range of areas, including virtual care delivery, digital health driven by wearables and connected medical devices, intelligent automation in administrative processes, enhanced cognitive capabilities in point-of-care decision systems, and bridging the payer and provider gap with drug manufacturers and therapeutic access through real-world data (Krittanawong, Zhang, & Wang, 2020).

While the potential for AI in healthcare is enormous, many barriers must be overcome for its successful adoption. Some of the main barriers include concerns about data privacy and security, the need for regulatory approval, the lack of standardization, and the cost of implementation (Takahashi et al., 2020). Moreover, cultural resistance to change and a lack of trust in AI technology could hinder its adoption. Therefore, it is essential to address these barriers and to create a supportive ecosystem that fosters innovation,

DOI: 10.1201/9781003262152-7

collaboration, and transparency in implementing AI in healthcare. This chapter provides an overview of the significant barriers to AI's application in healthcare and discusses strategies to overcome these barriers.

Barriers

While AI has emerged as a promising technology with the potential to transform the healthcare industry by enhancing clinical decision-making, improving patient outcomes, and reducing costs, the application of AI in healthcare faces various barriers that need to be addressed for its successful adoption. These barriers range from technical and regulatory challenges to cultural and ethical issues. Understanding and addressing these barriers is crucial for realizing the full potential of AI in healthcare.

Trust

Trust is one of the most significant barriers to the widespread adoption of AI in healthcare. AI in healthcare is hampered by a lack of trust among patients and healthcare professionals. Trust is an essential component of healthcare with or without AI. For AI systems, trust is particularly pertinent in healthcare because its reliability, safety, and security are assured before they can be used in clinical settings. A survey by EY found that 33% of US CEOs cite employee trust as one of the most significant barriers to AI adoption (EY, 2019). In the case of healthcare, trust is particularly critical because patients' lives are at stake, and the technology must be proven safe and effective before it can be widely adopted.

One of the main factors that can erode trust in AI systems is bias and model fairness. Bias can be introduced at various stages of the AI development process, from data collection to algorithm design and training. Biased AI systems can lead to health disparities, especially for underrepresented or underserved groups, and perpetuate existing inequalities in healthcare. Therefore, building the thoughtful implementations of AI that don't propagate the bias in that data is critical. Another concern is that AI systems may not be as accurate as human doctors. AI systems are trained on large datasets of medical data, but mistakes can still be made. For example, an AI system used to diagnose skin cancer was found to be less accurate than the performance of human dermatologists. Finally, some people are concerned that AI systems will replace human doctors. However, while AI systems can automate some tasks, they cannot replace human doctors. AI systems need to be trained and supervised by human doctors, and they cannot provide the same level of care.

Selection of Use Cases

AI has revolutionized the healthcare industry by offering various innovative solutions, from diagnostic algorithms to predictive models. However, the selection of the correct use cases is critical to ensuring that AI systems deliver safe and effective healthcare. The incorrect selection of use cases can introduce significant risks to patient safety and undermine the technology's credibility. One substantial risk associated with the wrong selection of use cases is the potential for algorithmic bias. Algorithms are trained on large datasets, and the algorithm can produce biased results if the dataset is biased. For instance, if an algorithm is trained on data that disproportionately represents a particular demographic group, such as middle-aged white men, the algorithm may produce inaccurate or discriminatory results when applied to other demographic groups. This can result in the misdiagnosis of conditions, leading to inappropriate treatments or delayed interventions, negatively impacting patient outcomes (Kagaya et al., 2018).

Another risk associated with the incorrect selection of use cases is the potential for inadequate data quality. AI algorithms require high-quality data to function accurately. If the data used to train the algorithm is incomplete, inaccurate, or outdated, the algorithm may produce incorrect or misleading results. This can lead to mistaken diagnoses or treatment plans, severely affecting patient health. Furthermore, if the AI system is not adequately validated and tested, it may not be reliable or safe for clinical use, introducing additional risks to patient safety.

Therefore, the selection of use cases in AI applications in healthcare is a critical factor in ensuring patient safety and the effectiveness of the technology. Healthcare providers and AI developers must consider the risks of selecting use cases, including algorithmic bias and data quality issues. Additionally, rigorous validation and testing of AI systems must be performed to ensure their reliability and safety in clinical settings (Topol, 2019).

Data

AI has the potential to revolutionize healthcare by improving diagnosis, treatment, and the prevention of disease. However, several challenges must be addressed before AI can be fully realized in healthcare. One of the biggest challenges is the volume of data required to train AI models. AI models need to be trained on large datasets of labelled data to learn how to make accurate predictions. This can be a challenge in healthcare because of the sensitive nature of patient data.

The amount of data that is generated in healthcare is increasing exponentially. In 2020, it was estimated that the healthcare industry generated 270 gigabytes of data for every person on Earth (RBC Capital Markets, n.d.). This data comes from a variety of sources, including electronic health records, medical devices, and wearables. This data is essential for training AI models, but it can also prove challenging to manage. The sheer volume of data can make storing, processing, and analyzing difficult. In addition, the data may be in different formats and not well-organized. This can make it difficult to extract insights from the data. Ensuring data interoperability is essential to guaranteeing data integrity fit for purpose. It means that data should be available, accessible, and shareable among different systems to support the interoperability of AI systems (Jiang et al., 2017).

Another challenge for AI in healthcare is privacy. The privacy component in AI systems has two branches: the privacy, security, and protection of the data needed to fuel AI and the confidentiality and security of deployed AI systems (Jiang et al., 2017). AI models are trained on data that is collected from patients. This data may include sensitive information, such as medical history, diagnoses, and treatment plans. It is essential to protect this data from unauthorized access. If this data were compromised, it could have severe consequences for patients. For example, their health information could be used to commit identity theft or to discriminate against them. Under emerging data privacy regulations such as GDPR and CCPA, working directly with personal data becomes extremely limited, and working with anonymized data is incredibly difficult and resource-intensive. Data de-identification, privacy-preserving AI, and federated data systems are among the measures that can be used to protect sensitive data while ensuring that AI systems comply with privacy regulations.

Biases

Algorithmic bias is defined as the application of an algorithm that compounds existing inequities in socioeconomic status, race, ethnic background, religion, gender, disability, or sexual orientation and amplifies inequities in health systems (Panch et al., 2019). Algorithmic bias is not a new issue and is not exclusive to AI. In healthcare, it can arise for a number of different factors, such as a lack of diversity in datasets used to develop algorithms, biased algorithms, or inappropriate application. The outcome of such biases can lead to inaccurate diagnoses, underdiagnosis, or overtreatment, which ultimately harms patients.

In the Framingham Heart Study, the cardiovascular risk score demonstrates one example of algorithmic bias in healthcare. The score performed well for Caucasian patients but not for African American ones, leading to the unequal distribution of care and inaccurate diagnoses. Similarly, studies in genomics and genetics have found that data collected for these studies are predominantly from Caucasians, making the studies less applicable to underrepresented groups (Panch et al., 2019).

Diabetic retinopathy (DR) is a severe complication of diabetes that can lead to vision loss, making early detection and timely intervention crucial for the prevention of blindness. Artificial Intelligence (AI) has shown potential in improving the accuracy and efficiency of DR screening. Gulshan et al. (2016) developed and validated a deep learning algorithm for detecting DR in retinal fundus photographs, demonstrating the potential of AI-based DR screening. However, the translation of AI-based DR screening systems into real-world clinical settings faces multiple challenges, including data quality and diversity, integration into existing healthcare systems, and regulatory and ethical considerations.

To address these challenges, it is essential to improve data quality and diversity by collaborating with researchers, healthcare providers, and patient advocacy groups to create more representative datasets (Gulshan et al., 2016). Additionally, techniques, such as data augmentation and transfer learning, can be employed to enhance algorithm performance. It is also crucial to enhance the integration of AI-based DR screening systems into existing clinical workflows by developing user-friendly interfaces, integrating them with electronic health record (EHR) systems, and providing education and training to healthcare providers. Ensuring adherence to data privacy regulations, implementing robust data security measures, and collaborating with regulatory bodies to obtain necessary approvals and certifications are vital to address regulatory and ethical concerns (Gulshan et al., 2016).

Overcoming these translational challenges can pave the way for the widespread adoption of AI-based DR screening and improve patient outcomes. The success of AI-based DR screening also has broader implications for the application of AI in healthcare, demonstrating that addressing these challenges can lead to more effective and efficient healthcare delivery (Gulshan et al., 2016).

The effects of algorithmic bias on patients can be far-reaching and damaging. Biased algorithms can perpetuate existing inequities and increase disparities in healthcare outcomes, leading to lower life expectancy and quality of life for particular groups (Powers, 2019). In addition, biased algorithms can result in incorrect diagnoses or treatment recommendations, leading to further health complications and potentially life-threatening situations.

Solutions and Opportunities

Artificial Intelligence (AI) in healthcare presents numerous opportunities for improving patient outcomes and streamlining processes. However, several challenges must be addressed to realize the full potential of AI in this domain. This chapter explores solutions for overcoming these challenges, including trust, selecting the correct use cases, data volume and privacy, bias in AI, and engaging healthcare workers.

Trust in AI in Healthcare

The first challenge in implementing AI in healthcare is establishing trust. Two main strategies can be employed to foster trust: education and explainability (Dataiku, 2020). Healthcare executives must ensure that individuals at all levels understand the basics of AI, making it more accessible and less intimidating. Most healthcare professionals below 40 already view digital health technologies as essential for better patient outcomes (Health IT Analytics, 2019). Moreover, AI systems must be a white box, meaning users are able to understand how they work and to interpret the results (Dataiku, 2020). This can be achieved by using explainability features and tools that combat bias, ensuring users understand model outputs and promoting trust and fairness.

Many healthcare workers are concerned about the potential impact of AI on employment (HIMSS, 2021). AI tools can increase the efficiency of many specialized jobs in the healthcare industry by taking over labour-intensive and repetitive procedures, freeing up clinicians' time for more complex tasks (Dilmegani, 2022a). To overcome this challenge, healthcare organizations should provide training to upskill their workers for AI and machine learning technologies and their applications. This will help organizations create a workforce that is confident in using emerging technologies and employees with their long-term careers.

Lastly, patient reluctance is a significant challenge in implementing AI in healthcare. People resist change and are more accepting of familiar things, especially regarding healthcare (Businesswire, 2020). For example, at the beginning of the COVID-19 pandemic, patients were uncomfortable with online checkups. However, now many people prefer it (Businesswire, 2020). Educating patients about the benefits of AI, such as reduced post-procedure pain and other complications, can help reduce hesitations and increase acceptance of AI-driven healthcare solutions.

Selecting the Right Use Cases

After establishing trust, the next step is selecting the appropriate use cases for AI in healthcare. Ideal AI projects should have clear answers to critical questions such as who will benefit, how the project will improve outcomes, why AI is better than existing processes, the upside and consequences of success or failure, data source, and the timeline for delivery. Some examples of healthcare use cases include staffing and resource planning, AI-assisted coding in medical claims billing, patient risk and care delivery models, and medical imaging classification (Dataiku, 2020).

Data

Finding high-quality medical data is another major challenge in implementing AI in healthcare. The sensitive nature and ethical constraints attached to medical data make it difficult to collect (Dilmegani, 2022a). Since annotating a single model can require about 10,000 images, this can cause the processing time-consuming and expensive, even when automated. New ways of medical image annotation are helping to overcome this challenge by extracting more data sets from one image and significantly reducing the amount of data needed to train a model (National Academies of Sciences, Engineering, and Medicine, 2015).

Compliance with data regulations is another significant challenge in healthcare AI. AI platforms can help by providing data cataloguing, access restriction and control, and minimization (Dataiku, 2020). However, the lack of labelled data for critical use cases, such as medical imaging, remains challenging. Organizations must have a data management system allowing data labelling to address this issue.

Several solutions can be used to address the challenges of data volume. One solution is to use AI to manage data. AI can automate tasks such as data collection, cleaning, and analysis. This can help to reduce the amount of manual work that is required to manage data. In addition, AI can be used to identify patterns in data that would not be visible to humans. This can help to extract insights from data that would otherwise be difficult to obtain.

Addressing Bias in AI

There is no simple solution to address algorithmic bias in healthcare. However, one strategy is to ensure that data science teams working on healthcare algorithms include professionals from diverse backgrounds and perspectives, not solely data scientists with technical expertise in AI (Panch et al., 2019). This approach helps to address the underlying values and societal norms that inform healthcare outcomes and reduce the influence of any single perspective.

Combating algorithmic bias requires data science teams to include diverse backgrounds and perspectives. Although this approach is unproven, technical solutions may also involve setting artificial standards in algorithms to emphasize disadvantaged groups and de-emphasize others. A tradeoff exists between performance and preference in algorithms, and addressing bias will necessitate collaboration between the private sector, government, academia, and civil society (Dataiku, 2020).

Privacy-Enhancing Technologies

The sensitive nature of patient data necessitates investment in privacy-enhancing technologies (PETs) to minimize the risk of data breaches while maximizing utility (Dilmegani, 2022b.). Traditional methods like data masking can be employed, along with emerging PETs such as differential privacy, homomorphic encryption, secure multi-party computation, and zero-knowledge proofs (Dilmegani, 2022b.). These techniques can train AI models without compromising patients' privacy. For example, differential privacy is a technique that can be used to add noise to data to protect individual privacy. This noise makes it difficult to identify individual patients, but it does not prevent the AI model from learning from the data.

Understanding AI Results and Testing AI

Healthcare workers must understand how and why AI produces specific results to ensure reliability and confidence in the technology. Explainable AI (XAI) methods can help justify AI-generated solutions, while thorough testing and verification can prevent diagnostic errors (National Academies Press, 2015). Healthcare organizations must ensure that training data is representative, and models generalize well without underfitting or overfitting (Dilmegani, 2022a).

Building AI Governance

The biggest challenges for AI in healthcare are not inherently technological; instead, they stem from people- and process-based issues (Health IT Analytics, 2019). To overcome these challenges, it is essential to build robust AI governance, develop innovative data annotation methods, train healthcare workers, and educate patients about the benefits of AI. AI governance is critical in breaking down barriers to AI adoption in healthcare. An AI governance framework enforces organizational priorities through standardized rules, processes, and requirements that shape how AI is designed, developed, and deployed (Dataiku, 2020). This kind of oversight can help build trust while ensuring data privacy, and, when implemented correctly, it can also foster flexibility that allows AI projects to thrive. Strong AI governance is necessary to make AI more accessible and user-friendly in healthcare. Developing a robust AI governance program can help address barriers in healthcare AI by enforcing standardized rules, processes, and requirements for AI design, development, and deployment (Dataiku, 2021). Another strategy is to prioritize the protection of disadvantaged groups by setting an artificial standard in the algorithm that overemphasizes these groups while de-emphasizing others. While this approach is technically challenging and unproven, it can potentially mitigate the harmful effects of algorithmic bias on these groups (Panch et al., 2019).

Overcoming the challenges of AI adoption in healthcare requires a multifaceted approach that includes strong AI governance, innovative data annotation methods,

TABLE 7.1

Translational Challenges of Application of AI in Healthcare and Their Solutions

Challenges	Solutions
1. AI Governance	Build a robust AI governance framework that enforces organizational priorities, rules, processes, and requirements.
2. Finding High-Quality Medical Data	Develop innovative data annotation methods to extract more data sets from one image and reduce data needed for training.
3. Perception of AI Among Healthcare Providers	Provide training and upskilling for healthcare workers in AI and machine learning technologies and their applications.
4. Patient Reluctance in Adopting AI-driven Healthcare	Educate patients about the benefits of AI to reduce hesitations and increase acceptance of AI-driven healthcare solutions.
5. Data Privacy and Security	Implement robust data protection measures and regulatory compliance to ensure patient data privacy and security.
6. Integration with Existing Systems	Create seamless integration between AI-driven tools and existing healthcare systems for better interoperability.
7. Ensuring Equity in AI Implementation	Develop AI systems that consider social determinants of health, avoid bias, and promote equitable healthcare outcomes.
8. Scalability and Adaptability of AI Solutions	Design AI-driven healthcare tools that are scalable and adaptable to different healthcare settings and contexts.
9. Trustworthiness of AI Algorithms	Employ white-box AI and transparent algorithms to build trust with end users and stakeholders.
10. Collaboration between AI Developers and Healthcare Professionals	Foster collaboration and communication between AI developers and healthcare professionals to align AI solutions with clinical needs.

Source: Authors.

training and education for healthcare workers, and patient education. By addressing these challenges, AI can be more effectively integrated into healthcare, ultimately improving patient outcomes and the healthcare system. Table 7.1 outlines the current translational challenges with the applications of AI in healthcare with accompanying solutions.

Conclusion

In conclusion, the adoption of AI in healthcare faces numerous challenges, from trust issues and data privacy concerns to the reluctance of patients and healthcare professionals. However, with proper education, training, and governance, these challenges can be addressed, allowing AI to revolutionize healthcare and improve patient outcomes. AI in healthcare is a complex and diverse field that can potentially transform the healthcare industry in many ways. It is essential to recognize that AI is not meant to replace physicians but to assist them in making more informed decisions and improving patient outcomes. However, to fully realize the potential of AI in healthcare, there is a need to address the existing barriers and challenges and create a supportive environment that fosters innovation and collaboration.

References

Businesswire. (2020). Patients prefer physicians who offer telemedicine during COVID-19 and beyond, says new everyday health and klick health research. Retrieved April 30, 2023, from https://www.businesswire.com/news/home/20200806005248/en/

Dataiku. (2020). White-box vs. black-box models: Balancing interpretability and accuracy. Retrieved April 30, 2023, from https://blog.dataiku.com/white-box-vs-black-box-models-balancing-interpretability-and-accuracy

Dataiku. (2021). Model interpretability. Retrieved April 30, 2023, from https://blog.dataiku.com/model-interpretability

Dilmegani, C. (2022a). Examples of AI project failures. *AI Multiple*. Retrieved April 30, 2023, from https://research.aimultiple.com/ai-fail/#what-are-some-examples-of-ai-project-failures

Dilmegani, C. (2022b). Top 10 privacy enhancing technologies & use cases in 2023. *AI Multiple*. Retrieved April 30, 2023, from https://research.aimultiple.com/privacy-enhancing-technologies/

EY. (2019). The AI race: Barriers, opportunities, and optimism. Retrieved April 30, 2023, from https://assets.ey.com/content/dam/ey-sites/ey-com/en_gl/news/2019/05/ey-the-ai-race-barriers-opportunities-and-optimism.pdf

Gulshan, V., Peng, L., Coram, M., Stumpe, M. C., Wu, D., Narayanaswamy, A., ... & Webster, D. R. (2016). Development and validation of a deep learning algorithm for detection of diabetic retinopathy in retinal fundus photographs. *JAMA*, 316(22), 2402–2410. doi:10.1001/jama.2016.17216

Health IT Analytics. (2019). One-third of young providers overwhelmed by patient data analytics. Retrieved April 30, 2023, from https://healthitanalytics.com/news/one-third-of-young-providers-overwhelmed-by-patient-data-analytics

HIMSS. (2021). State of healthcare report: Uncovering healthcare barriers and opportunities. Retrieved April 30, 2023, from https://www.himss.org/resources/state-healthcare-report-uncovering-healthcare-barriers-and-opportunities

Jiang, F., Jiang, Y., Zhi, H., et al. (2017). Artificial intelligence in healthcare: Past, present and future. *Stroke and Vascular Neurology*, 2, doi:10.1136/svn-2017-000101

Kagaya, H. R., Li, Z., Li, Q., Liu, H., & Zhang, J. (2018). Bias in healthcare artificial intelligence: The need for diversity and data governance in machine learning. *Technology in Society*, 55, 100–105. doi:10.1016/j.techsoc.2018.06.001

Krittanawong, C., Zhang, H., & Wang, Z. (2020). Artificial intelligence in precision cardiovascular medicine. *Journal of the American College of Cardiology*, 75(23), 2985–2997. doi:10.1016/j.jacc.2020.04.040

National Academies of Sciences, Engineering, and Medicine. (2015). *Improving diagnosis in healthcare*. The National Academies Press. https://www.nap.edu/catalog/21794/improving-diagnosis-in-health-care

Panch, T., Mattie, H., & Atun, R. (2019). Artificial intelligence and algorithmic bias: Implications for health systems. *Journal of Global Health*, 9(2), 1–7. https://www.ncbi.nlm.nih.gov/pmc/articles/PMC6875681/

Powers, B. (2019). Racial bias in health care algorithms. *Science*, 366(6464), 447–448. doi:10.1126/science.aaz8289

RBC Capital Markets. (n.d.). The healthcare data explosion. Retrieved April 30, 2023, from https://www.rbccm.com/en/gib/healthcare/episode/the_healthcare_data_explosion

Takahashi, Y., Sakamoto, N., Iwata, S., Mori, Y., Ishikawa, H., Matsumura, Y., ... & Takeda, T. (2020). Adoption of artificial intelligence in healthcare. *Lancet Digital Health*, 2(10), e484–e486. doi:10.1016/s2589-7500(20)30181-5

Topol, E. J. (2019). High-performance medicine: The convergence of human and artificial intelligence. *Nature Medicine*, 25(1), 44–56. doi:10.1038/s41591-018-0300-7

8

The Translational Application of AI in Healthcare

Piyush Mathur and Francis Papay
Cleveland Clinic, Cleveland, OH, USA

LEARNING OBJECTIVES

- Learn about how AI is currently implemented in healthcare.
- Describe methods to evaluate the successful implementation of AI in healthcare.
- Identify the pitfalls and challenges related to the implementation of AI in healthcare.

Introduction

Since the Food and Drug Administration (FDA) approved the first artificial intelligence (AI) diagnostic solution for the detection of diabetic retinopathy in 2018, there has been a rapid proliferation of AI-based devices being approved for implementation and use at the bedside (Hand, 2018). The exponential growth in research has preceded the development of these AI solutions, which are beginning to be introduced after validation trials. An ever-increasing amount of innovation in the AI models, the adoption of cloud computing, the implementation of electronic health records (EHRs), and the availability of non-EHR data (sensor data, social media data) have translated into exponential progress in research related to AI in healthcare. In recent years, we are finding that this research in healthcare follows AI's evolution, from the use of structured data elements and image analysis to, more recently, the use of large language models.

Both the quantity and the quality of research have also increased and improved, leading to more mature publications across the healthcare spectrum (Zhang et al., 2022). The mature stage of such AI publication was identified as studies involving research that tests an AI model against a real-world gold standard, or in real-world evaluation.

DOI: 10.1201/9781003262152-8

According to an analysis by Zhang et al., areas of healthcare such as respiratory medicine and the treatment of breast cancer and retinopathy demonstrate the greatest production of mature research relative to total research production (Zhang et al., 2022). The distribution of multimodal data types of usage across major subspecialties has also grown across all specialties. Clearly, there are leading areas, such as radiology, ophthalmology, oncology, and cardiology, among the healthcare specialties, especially those that have benefited from the availability of data, such as imaging data. More recently, multimodal approaches using a combination of text, image, and/or audio data are being used in the research and development of AI solutions that mimic a clinician more than the older narrow-spectrum AI development (Acosta, Falcone, Rajpurkar, & Topol, 2022).

New and evolving fields, such as radiomics and pathomics, are currently laying the foundation for the next generation of AI-guided laboratory and imaging diagnostics. The term "radiomics" refers to the extraction of mineable data from medical imaging and has been applied within oncology to improve diagnosis, prognostication, and clinical decision support, with the goal of delivering precision medicine. Since it was first coined in 2012, the term "radiomics" in the literature has experienced an exponential increase, accounting for over 1,500 publications in 2020 alone (Shur et al., 2021). Similarly, the term "pathomics" refers to machine-learning methods and AI-based image analysis of tissues based on the identification and classification of tissue, architectural elements, cells, nuclei, and other histologic features used to study several types and subtypes of cancer (Gupta, Kurc, Sharma, Almeida, & Saltz, 2019). This term is seeing similar exponential growth in research and solutions development.

Additionally, within the healthcare sector, AI-guided drug development has been a large focus of the industry. The diverse range of AI applications being explored could help tackle the fundamental challenge of developing new drugs, from target identification through clinical trials, which typically require years of time and billions of dollars. Pharmaceutical companies are building their own in-house AI teams, as well as investing in and collaborating with these companies to develop more effective targeted drugs or repurpose molecules more efficiently. Previously, it may have taken the traditional drug discovery process around four or five years; the use of AI has significantly reduced this timeframe. For example, an A2 receptor antagonist designed to help T cells fight solid tumors was found in eight months through the harnessing of an AI design platform; this process would have otherwise taken many years. Knowing that 90 percent of candidate therapies fail somewhere between phase one trials and regulatory approval, the large, estimated price tag of USD 2.6 billion for developing a treatment can be reduced significantly (Fleming, 2018). Accelerated by ground-breaking research, the computational predictions of protein structure now approach the quality of those provided by gold-standard experimental techniques, such as X-ray crystallography, can be achieved (Callaway, 2020). Henstock cited projections indicating that the pharmaceutical industry could boost earnings by more than 45% by making strong investments in AI (Henstock, 2019).

CASE STUDY 1   EARLY ADOPTION OF DEEP LEARNING IN HEALTHCARE (MADANI, ARNAOUT, MOFRAD, & ARNAOUT, 2018)

INTRODUCTION

AI implementation in echocardiography is an example of the successful implementation of a data-rich, image-based study which usually requires highly trained and skilled clinicians to perform and interpret.

AI INTERVENTION

Through the use of the convolutional neural network (CNN), Madani et al. (2018) trained a model to simultaneously classify 15 standard views (12 video, 3 still), based on labelled still images and videos from 267 transthoracic echocardiograms that captured a range of real-world clinical variation.

RESULTS

Their model, incorporating 12 video views, performed with 97.8% overall test accuracy. Even on single low-resolution images, accuracy among 15 views was 91.7% compared with 70.2–84.0% for board-certified echocardiographers.

KEY POINT

Following early after successful demonstration of image classifiers using deep learning in 2012, researchers rapidly and successfully adopted similar modeling techniques for complex cardiac testing such as Echocardiography.

With an increasing number of submissions of the AI-based solution for regulatory approval, the FDA put forward a framework to facilitate innovation through AI medical-based solutions while providing the appropriate oversight and regulatory structure. In a study of governmental and non-governmental databases to identify AI-based devices, between 2015 and 2020 some 222 devices were approved for use in the USA and some 240 devices in Europe (Muehlematter, Daniore, & Vokinger, 2021). The majority of the AI/ML-based medical devices were approved for radiology (129 [58%]), followed by cardiovascular (40 [18%]) and neurological devices (21 [9%]). Interestingly, in the same analysis, it was found that the majority of the 172 (77%) AI/ML-based medical devices were marketed by small companies and only 50 (23%) by big companies. Most manufacturers were based in the USA (126 [57%] of 222 devices), followed by Israel (16 devices [7%]), and the rest from a large number of European countries. Of the 222 FDA-approved medical devices, 189 (85%) were intended for use by healthcare professionals, whereas 33 (15%) were intended for use directly by the patient.

Healthcare specialties, such as gastroenterology, anesthesiology, and critical care, are also learning from other specialties, utilizing new techniques and, in many instances, leapfrogging their research and development efforts over some of the key leading health-care specialties. The development and implementation of solutions, such as AI-guided colonoscopy, hypotension prediction index, and sepsis models, are key examples of how some of these specialties have developed, validated, and implemented AI in their clinical domains.

The Current State of AI Implementation in Healthcare

Moving beyond research and validation, it is encouraging to see phases of the early implementation of AI in healthcare. In the past, many have described the implementation of AI in healthcare along the categories of diagnostics, therapeutics, population management, and administration (He et al., 2019). We take a similar approach in reviewing the current state of the implementation of AI in healthcare.

Diagnostics

There are numerous examples of diagnosis generation or triage using patient-reported symptoms, sometimes combined with vital signs. To enable this, many have developed chatbots that collect patient information and use machine learning to generate diagnoses. In a review of 11 chatbot applications, You and Gui (2020) found that most of these applications can support five diagnostic processes that are included in the common offline medical encounter: collecting patient history, evaluating symptoms, prompting an initial diagnosis, suggesting diagnostic tests, and referrals or other follow-up treatments (You & Gui, 2020). Although promising, their review and analysis found that users found weaknesses in the following functions of these applications: health history data collection, symptoms input, detailed questions regarding presentation, medication information, and user group support. The authors concluded that the future conversational design of healthcare chatbots should consider how to improve input flexibility, including a design to assist users in inputting their symptoms and the ability to ask detailed questions with explainability features. Amongst the key areas of image-based diagnostics have been radiology-diagnosing AI algorithms, such as the diagnosis of acute stroke, large vessel occlusion, acute pulmonary embolism, pulmonary nodules, and aortic dissection from MRI or CT scans.

In a review of five commercially available software platforms, their applications, and related publications, the researchers summarized the current state of stroke imaging using AI (Soun et al., 2021). A computer-automated detection (CAD) algorithm on non-contrast head CT scans to detect subtle changes in attenuation in patients with ischemic stroke improved the detection of strokes for emergency physicians and radiology residents (an AUC of 0.879 improved to 0.942 for emergency physicians, and an AUC of 0.965 improved to 0.990 for radiology residents) (Tang, Ng, & Chow, 2011). When trialled with experienced radiologists, however, it did not significantly improve stroke detection as there were already high stroke detection rates. Another study showed that an artificial neural network (ANN) was able to distinguish acute stroke within 4.5 hours of onset (which was verified by clinical and CT and MR imaging data) with a mean sensitivity of 80.0% and specificity of 86.2% (Abedi et al., 2017). Going further, since infarct volumes are important to triage patients for appropriate therapy, AI has been able to establish core infarct volumes through automatic lesion segmentation. The largest cohort based on an ANN was able to identify core infarct volume with an AUC of 0.85 (Kasasbeh et al., 2019).

From a therapeutics perspective, in an acute ischemic stroke, diagnosing large vessel occlusion (LVO) is essential for identifying candidates who could benefit from mechanical thrombectomy. A CNN-based commercial software detected proximal LVO with an AUC of 86%, helping with the triage of stroke patients (Chatterjee, Somayaji, & Kabakis, 2019). Prognostication is also an important aspect of managing these patients with acute strokes. Soun et al. (2021) summarized how the current state of various machine learning (ML) algorithms had been used to predict imaging and clinical outcomes after ischemic stroke. One of the commercially available software programs was able to predict poor clinical outcomes after thrombectomy and was an independent predictor of poor outcomes in multivariate analysis (OR, 0.79; 95% CI, 0.63–0.99). Traditional ML techniques combining clinical data and the core–penumbra mismatch ratio derived from MR imaging and MRP to determine post-thrombolysis clinical outcomes performed with an AUC of 0.863 (95%) for short-term (day 7) outcomes and 0.778 (95%) for long-term (day 90) outcomes. Decision-tree-based algorithms using extreme gradient boosting and gradient boosting machines were able to predict a 90-day modified Rankin scale (mRS) > 2 using combined imaging and clinical data with an AUC of 0.74. Similar results, especially with additional clinical data post-intervention for large vessel occlusion, have been found using neural networks in many other studies. Finally, traditional ML techniques and neural networks were used to predict significant complications, such as the hemorrhagic transformation of acute ischemic stroke before treatment from MRI images, with the highest AUC of 0.83.

AI for intracranial hemorrhage has gained one of the most rapid implementations across healthcare, largely due to the availability of data from which deep learning algorithms can be built. One of the largest cohorts for the detection and classification of intracranial hemorrhage (ICH) examined more than 30,0000 non-contrast CT (NCCTs) of heads from different hospitals in India using DL algorithms. The algorithm performed well on two different validation datasets, achieving AUCs of 0.92 and 0.94, respectively, for detecting ICH (Chilamkurthy et al., 2018). Diagnosing the type of hemorrhage is very important for clinical management. These algorithms are also able to classify subtypes of hemorrhage, such as parenchymal, intraventricular, subdural, extradural/epidural, and subarachnoid, with AUCs ranging from 0.90 to 0.97. ICH quantification using these deep learning algorithms achieved significant correlation Pearson correlation coefficients (0.953–0.999) for various types of hemorrhages when compared with semiautomated segmentation by a radiologist in the real-life prospective testing of the algorithm.

The study of aortic diseases is seeing an increasing number of investigations using deep learning methods, including strategies to screen the presence of aortic dissection on CT scans, automatically segment CT datasets with aortic dissection, and combine clinical and imaging variables to improve risk prediction (Mastrodicasa et al., 2022). AI has been heavily researched for early detection and characterizing lung nodules and for guiding prognostic assessment. This research has included the development of AI tools for image post-processing (e.g., the vessel suppression on CT) and for noninterpretive aspects of reporting and workflow, including management of nodule follow-up. Despite all this research and the FDA approval of AI tools for pulmonary nodule evaluation, integration into clinical practice has been challenging. Challenges to clinical adoption have included concerns about generalizability, technical hurdles in implementation, and concerns about bias (Liu, Yang, & Tsai, 2022).

Similar to image-oriented deep learning solutions for radiology, for histopathological diagnosis, solutions have been developed to leverage AI-based feature engineering for the assessment of NASH cirrhosis and tumour or lymphoid structures from tissue biopsies. The digitization of whole slide images (WSI) has accelerated the availability of data, ready for deep learning solutions to be applied.

There are currently several virtual microscope applications that facilitate the visualization of WSIs for pathomics analyses that include open-source and commercial software tools for WSIs. These software applications assist with data collection, annotation, and application of deep learning pathetic solutions, such as nuclear segmentation, tumour identification, and lymphocyte detection. According to Gupta et al. (2019), the increasing availability of data is set to turn the collective insight into cancer and provide pathologists with tools that will allow them to interpret their visual inspection in unprecedented ways. Various examples in current development include artificial-intelligence-powered immune phenotyping of urothelial carcinoma WSIs, a machine learning model to identify tertiary lymphoid structures in histopathological images, and a machine learning prediction of the NASH fibrosis stage without manual annotation.

AI-guided non-radiology-image-based diagnosis also includes endoscopy, retinal fundus evaluation, and echocardiography, which are now in use in clinical areas.

Many solutions now use multimodal solutions integrating data from imaging, laboratory tests, and text data, among others, to generate a diagnosis.

AI techniques based on deep learning algorithms can assist endoscopists in detecting lesions in intestines and identify benign vs malignant lesions and those requiring biopsy. Computer-aided detection (CADe) has been associated with an increase in small and large bowel adenoma detection rates, a key quality metric for gastroenterologists performing endoscopy. Over the past few years, 50 randomized controlled trials, comprising 34,445 participants, were included in an analysis of a systematic review and a meta-analysis performed by Spadaccini et al. (2021) (six trials of CADe, 18 of chromoendoscopy, and 26 of increased mucosal visualization systems). Compared with the control technique of HD white-light endoscopy, the adenoma detection rate was 7.4% higher with CADe, 4.4% higher with chromoendoscopy, and 4.1% higher with increased mucosal visualization systems. When focusing on large adenomas (≥10 mm), there was a significant increase in the detection of large adenomas only with CADe when compared to HD white-light endoscopy. CADe also seemed to be the superior strategy for the detection of sessile serrated lesions. No significant difference in the scope withdrawal time was reported for CADe compared with the other techniques. Hence, there is growing support for the wider incorporation of CADe strategies into endoscopy services across the world.

Automated electrocardiogram (ECG) interpretation has been in clinical use for many decades. AI, especially with the incorporation of optical sensors on wearable devices that can detect irregular pulses to identify atrial fibrillation during typical use, has grown in use. In a recently conducted study of 419,297 participants conducted over eight months, 2161 participants (0.52%) received notifications of an irregular pulse (Perez et al., 2019). Among the 450 participants who returned ECG patches that could be analyzed, atrial fibrillation was present in over 34% of the participants. Among participants who were notified of an irregular pulse, the positive predictive value was 0.84 (95% CI, 0.76 to 0.92) for observing atrial fibrillation.

ECG-based diagnosis of other cardiac conditions, such as heart failure (low EF prediction), is also being researched. A deep learning algorithm to detect low ejection fraction (EF) using a routine 12-lead electrocardiogram (ECG) has recently been developed and validated (Yao et al., 2020). The algorithm was incorporated into the electronic health record (EHR) to automatically screen for low EF and prospectively evaluate a novel artificial intelligence (AI) screening tool for detecting low EF in primary care practices. Furthermore, trials of this deep learning algorithm will examine the effectiveness of the AI-enabled ECG for the detection of asymptomatic low EF in routine primary care practices.

Similar to ECG, echocardiography is a uniquely well-suited approach for the application of deep learning in cardiology, critical care, and many other healthcare specialties which have adopted echocardiography as a point-of-care device. For diagnoses ranging from ischemic or non-ischemic cardiomyopathies to valvular heart diseases, echocardiography is essential. But there is evidence of variance in the human interpretation of echocardiogram images that could impact clinical care even amongst the trained cardiologists, despite guidelines. Researchers using convolutional neural networks on a large dataset showed that deep learning could be applied to echocardiography to identify local cardiac structures, estimate cardiac function, and predict systemic phenotypes that modify cardiovascular risk but are not readily identifiable to human interpretation (Ghorbani et al., 2020). Their deep learning model trained on a data set of more than 2.6 million echocardiogram images from 2850 patients, EchoNet (Figure 8.1), accurately identified the presence of pacemaker leads (AUC = 0.89), enlarged left atriums (AUC = 0.86), left ventricular hypertrophies (AUC = 0.75), left ventricular end-systolic and diastolic volumes ($R^2 = 0.74$ and $R^2 = 0.70$), and ejection fractions ($R^2 = 0.50$), as well as predicting systemic phenotypes of age ($R^2 = 0.46$), sex (AUC = 0.88), weight ($R^2 = 0.56$), and height ($R^2 = 0.33$). They concluded that the use of deep learning on echocardiography images could streamline repetitive tasks in the clinical workflow, provide preliminary interpretation in areas with insufficient qualified cardiologists, and predict phenotypes challenging for human evaluation.

A. EchoNet workflow for image selection, cleaning, and model training. B. Comparison of model performance with different cardiac views as input. C. Examples of data augmentation. The original frame is rotated (left to right) and its intensity is increase (top to bottom) as augmentation.

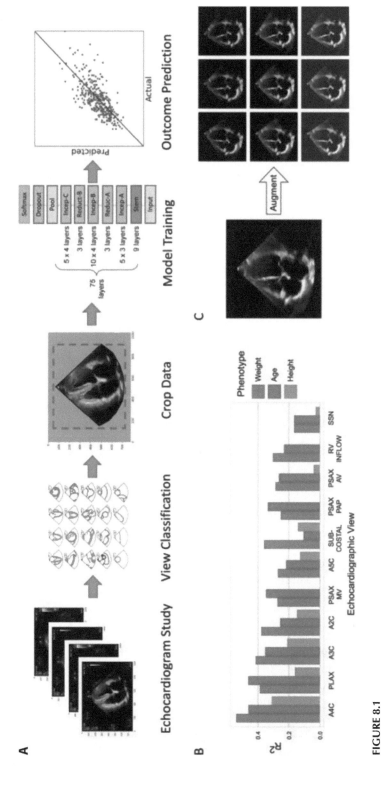

FIGURE 8.1

EchoNet machine learning pipeline for outcome prediction.

(Source: Ghorbani et al., 2020.)

CASE STUDY 2   FEASIBILITY AND UTILITY STUDIES FOR AI-BASED ECHOCARDIOGRAPHY IN HEALTHCARE (NARANG ET AL., 2021)

INTRODUCTION

After the successful development of datasets and the development of deep learning models, additional evaluation of implementation of AI-based echocardiography has followed.

AI INTERVENTION

Prospective, multicenter diagnostic study was conducted at two academic hospitals with a cohort of eight nurses who had not previously conducted echocardiograms. Each patient underwent paired limited echocardiograms: one from a nurse without prior echocardiography experience were instructed to obtain ten standard TTE views using the DL algorithm and the other from a sonographer without the DL algorithm.

RESULTS

When the studies were reviewed by a blind study, expert echocardiographers, there was an agreement of greater than 90% between the nurse-acquired and sonographer-acquired studies when adjudicating whether LV size (95.7%), LV function (96.6%), RV size (92.5%), RV function (92.9%), presence of a nontrivial pericardial effusion (99.6%), aortic valve structure (90.6%), mitral valve structure (93.3%), and tricuspid valve structure (95.2%) were deemed either normal/borderline or abnormal.

KEY POINT

Beyond demonstrating the accuracy of AI model for its performance on classification task, its embedding in clinical devices and the assessment of its ease of use and successful utilization studies are important. Democratization of a key skill set such as echocardiography for image capture and its automated interpretation demonstrates the feasibility and utility of AI-based techniques in this clinical setting.

AI has been increasingly applied to dermatology since its early applications in the diagnosis of types of skin lesions from images. In a recent review of the literature, they found that most of the AI applications focused on differentiating between benign and malignant skin lesions; however, others exist pertaining to ulcers, inflammatory skin diseases, allergen exposure, dermatopathology, and gene expression profiling (Safran et al., 2018). To date, the greatest progress has taken place in the field of melanoma diagnosis, followed by ulcer and psoriasis assessment tools, and then numerous less frequently studied applications. Beyond the identification of skin lesions, many of these applications also use tools such as risk assessment calculators to ascertain the risk of disease progression. The authors have identified important barriers to implementation, including systematic biases, the difficulty of standardization, interpretability, and acceptance by physicians and patients alike. In a recent international survey of 1,271 dermatologists, 85.1% of responders were aware of AI as an emerging topic in their field, yet only 23.8% had good or excellent knowledge of the subject. Additionally, 77.3% agreed that AI would improve dermatological care, and 79.8% thought that AI should be part of medical training (Polesie et al., 2020).

In a recent review of melanoma screening applications, it was found that when dermatologists were involved in the study design, the AI applications leveraged significantly larger patient datasets that were more representative of true clinical scenarios (Zakhem, Fakhoury, Motosko, & Ho, 2021). While identifying similar barriers to the adoption of AI in dermatology, another group of researchers concluded that there is a larger need for clinical trials providing evidence of clinical efficacy while successfully overcoming the identified barriers (Gomolin, Netchiporouk, Gniadecki, & Litvinov, 2020).

With the availability of multimodal data, AI applications to diagnose and manage mental health have been evolving rapidly over the past few years. In a review of 28 studies of AI and mental health, EHRs data, mood rating scales, brain imaging data, novel monitoring systems (e.g., smartphone, video), and social media platforms were used to predict, classify, or subgroup mental health illnesses, including depression, schizophrenia, other psychiatric illnesses, and suicide ideation or attempts (Graham et al., 2019). These studies provided excellent examples of AI's potential in mental healthcare, but most should be considered early proof-of-concept applications, which did have a high degree of accuracy. They concluded that as researchers and practitioners vested in improving mental healthcare, we must take an active role in informing the introduction of AI into clinical care by lending our clinical expertise and collaborating with data and computational scientists, as well as other experts, to help transform mental health practice and improve care for patients.

Therapeutics

AI application for drug discovery has seen a high level of investment and innovation. Many companies are focusing on identifying molecular candidates and matching them with the disease states. These techniques not only accelerate the screening process for drug discovery but also help with more efficient clinical trial management. Commercial solutions have been developed that aim to treat neuropsychiatric disorders using multimodal data, which can phenotype patients better and increase the chances of successful drug development using machine-learning algorithms. Similarly, commercial applications are being developed that utilize AI and robotics to precisely treat cancerous tumours. The technology lets providers personalize stereotactic radiosurgery and stereotactic body radiation therapy for each patient. Virtual reality with AI-enabled devices permits surgeons to explore the patient's anatomy in detail and plan for complex surgical procedures in advance. Similar applications combining augmented reality and AI are currently being trialled and are available for commercial use for acute pain management, sedation for surgical procedures, the treatment of mental health disorders, and physical rehabilitation.

Administration

With the evolution of large health systems and organizations that treat millions of patients, report quality metrics, and require operations at scale, AI is being researched and adopted to assist with critical decision-making processes. Platforms such as these can help clinicians manage patients with chronic health conditions such as hypertension and diabetes, especially using device inputs, even remotely. Personalized healthcare plans can also be constructed using AI within the populations. Patient experience is being analyzed using AI, which can not only help with the assessment of patient comments but also look at wait times and utilization. Automations such as scheduling, billing, and claims management using a combination of robotic process automation and AI have made revenue cycle management easier. Commercially available solutions combine Big Data and AI to predict clinical, financial, and operational risk by taking data from existing sources; such predictions include identifying high-risk patients and measuring costs and efficiency. Applications using clinical and operational data are being adopted to predict ICU transfers, improve clinical workflows, determine a patient's risk of hospital-acquired infections, and ensure adherence to clinical care paths. Many AI tools are also being currently researched and implemented to aid administrative tasks, such as clinical note generation (speech to text), patient scheduling, patient triage, and building financial models.

Regulation Related to AI Implementation in Healthcare

A key element to implementing AI technologies in healthcare is the development of regulatory standards for the assessment of safety and efficacy. A voluntary group of medical device regulators working towards harmonizing international medical device regulation is the International Medical Device Regulators Forum (IMDRF), which defines SaMD (software as a medical device) as "software intended to be used for one or more medical purposes that perform these purposes without being part of a hardware medical device," and the US Food and Drug Administration (FDA) has put forth the Digital Health Innovation Action Plan, which outlines its approach to SaMD, including the use of AI technologies. The current process of approval of conventional medical device approvals in the United States, which goes through the FDA's Center for Devices and Radiological Health (CDRH), is not well suited for fast-paced cycles of iterative modification, which is what software entails. Hence, the FDA has developed and continues to develop a wide range of regulatory guidelines and discussion papers on the safety and ethics of AI systems (termed SaMD) in collaboration with other stakeholders. The FDA has also developed a Software Precertification Program, a "more streamlined and efficient" voluntary pathway, resulting in improved access to technologies. Similar to the FDA approach, IMDRF also recommends a continuous iterative process based on real-world performance data, and low-risk SaMD may not require independent review.

CASE STUDY 3   REGULATORY APPROVALS AND BEDSIDE IMPLEMENTATION

INTRODUCTION

Following development and validation of deep learning techniques, it has been important to follow evaluation frameworks, and obtain regulatory approvals to implement AI algorithms in clinical workspace

AI INTERVENTION

Evaluation of the AI-based algorithms and regulatory approval following guidance, like those provided by the agencies such as the FDA is an important step towards implementation in clinical settings.

RESULTS

There are multiple FDA-approved, commercially available, AI-guided echocardiography devices currently available and in clinical use.

KEY POINT

Principles as described in the application of Good Machine Learning (GMLP) provide guidance for the development and validation of AI algorithms for clinical settings.

Source: Good Machine Learning Practice for Medical Device Development: Guiding Principles. (2021, 10/27/2021). Retrieved from https://www.fda.gov/medical-devices/software-medical-device-samd/good-machine-learning-practice-medical-device-development-guiding-principles.

In an analysis of 137 AI-based devices, 59 FDA approvals were for 49 unique devices. These devices commonly assisted with diagnostic ($n = 35$) and triage ($n = 10$) tasks. Of these, 23 devices were assistive, providing decision support; 12 were automated in the provision of information to the clinician (e.g., estimation of cardiac ejection fraction); and 14 automatically provided task decisions such as triaging and the reading of scans according to suspected findings of stroke. The stages of human information processing that were the most automated by devices included information analysis ($n = 14$), providing analyzed information for clinician decision-making, and decision selection ($n = 29$), providing options for the clinician to make a decision (Chen, Lyell, Laranjo, & Magrabi, 2020).

Many other US government agencies are forming legislation that might impact the adoption of healthcare AI, such as the 21st Century Cures Act, related amendments to the Social Security Act, and the formation of the National Artificial Intelligence Advisory Committee (NAIAC). The National Committee of Quality Assurance (NCQA) can create or update new quality measures, described as the Healthcare Effectiveness Data and Information Set (HEDIS), with financial incentives tied to meeting a HEDIS measure for payors and providers. The United States Preventative Services Task Force (USPSTF) makes evidence-based recommendations about preventative services, which may include AI, that can affect patient access.

The European Union (EU) has issued some key regulatory policies that will affect AI implementation in their healthcare systems. The General Data Protection and Regulation (GDPR) outlined a comprehensive set of regulations for the collection, storage, and use of personal information, as adopted by the European Parliament in April 2016 and became effective in May 2018. A critical component of this regulation is Article 22, "Automated individual decision making, including profiling." This article of regulation describes the right of citizens to receive an explanation for algorithmic decisions. The GDPR will affect AI implementation in healthcare in several ways. First, it requires explicit and informed consent before any collection of personal data. Second, the new regulation essentially lends power to the person providing the data to track what data is being collected and to request the removal of their data. Finally, the need for a "right to explanation" will potentially limit the types of models that manufacturers can use in health-related applications. This is because, given the high stakes of dealing with human health, model interpretability is important in AI-based healthcare applications, and this requirement may actually help AI applications become more reliable and trustable while holding the manufacturers of AI-based technologies more accountable.

As in hospitals in the US and Europe, AI-based screening tools have already been deployed in clinical trials in multiple Chinese hospitals. In June 2019, China's regulatory body for life sciences products, the National Medical Product Administration (NMPA), issued "Technical Guideline on AI-Aided Software," which is similar to the FDA guidance. In 2020, the NMPA approved DeepVessel FFR, the first Class III "AImedical device to perform a physiological functional assessment of the coronary arteries noninvasively. It extracts three-dimensional coronary tree structures and computes fractional flow reserve (FFR) values in minutes from the coronary computed tomography angiography (CTA) scan.

Patients and patient organizations are also focusing efforts on providing inputs to the development of regulation and advocating patients' rights. For example, the American Diabetic Association (ADA) updated its standards of medical care for diabetes, and it supports the use of autonomous AI for diabetic retinal exams. The ADA has been involved in the comment process for the rules proposed by the US Centers for Medicare & Medicaid Services (CMS), as well as in the FDA's regulatory processes through the Patient Preference Initiative and other related guidance.

Revenue and Funding for Sustainable AI in Healthcare

Beyond the approval of AI algorithms for clinical adoptions by various regulatory bodies across the world, approval for reimbursement for the use of these applications is an important step for sustainable implementation. At its September 2021 meeting, the American Medical Association's (AMA) CPT® Editorial Panel accepted the addition of

TABLE 8.1

CPT Classification of AI Algorithms

Classification	Work Performed by AI/ML	Application Example (CPT Code)
Assistive	Machine **detects** clinically relevant data	Computer-aided detection (CAD) imaging(77065-77067)
Augmentative	Machine **analyzes** and/or **quantifies** data	Continuous glucose monitoring (CGM) (95251)
Autonomous	Machine **automatically interprets** data	Retinal imaging (92229)

Source: CMS, 2022

a new Appendix S to provide guidance for classifying various artificial intelligence/ augmented intelligence (AI) applications that describe work associated with the use of AI-enabled medical services and/or procedures for reimbursement (Source: American Medical Association, 2022).

There are three categories for AI applications per the guidelines, including assistive, augmentative, or autonomous (Table 8.1). This classification is based on the clinical procedure or service provided to the patient and the work performed by the machine on behalf of the clinician.

Assistive Classification

The work performed by the machine for the clinician is assistive when the machine detects clinically relevant data without analysis or generated conclusions. This requires clinician interpretation and report.

Augmentative Classification

The work performed by the machine for the clinician is augmentative when the machine analyzes and/or quantifies data in a clinically meaningful way. This requires a clinician and report.

Autonomous Classification

The work performed by the machine for the clinician is autonomous when the machine automatically interprets data and independently generates clinically meaningful conclusions without a concurrent physician or other QHP involvement. Autonomous medical services and procedures include interrogating and analyzing data. The work of the algorithm may or may not include the acquisition, preparation, and/or transmission of data. The clinically meaningful conclusion may be a characterization of data (e.g., the likelihood of pathophysiology) to be used to establish a diagnosis or to implement a therapeutic intervention. There are three further levels of autonomous AI medical services and procedures with varying levels and degrees of clinician involvement, graded based on offering diagnosis and management options to initiating management, which can be contested by a clinician.

The US Centers for Medicare and Medicaid Services (CMS), for the first time, established a national payment amount for an FDA *de novo* authorized autonomous AI system, in both the Medicare Physician Fee Schedule (MPFS) and the Outpatient Prospective

Payment System (OPPS), for IDx-DR system (Digital Diagnostics, Coralville, Iowa, USA). This autonomous AI system makes a clinical decision without human oversight and diagnoses a specific disease, as described by its new CPT® code 92229. CMS also, for the first time, established a national add-on payment for assistive AI under the New Technology Add-on Payments (NTAP) in the Inpatient Prospective Payment System (IPPS) for the Viz LVO system for stroke detection and the Caption Guidance system for cardiac ultrasound to enable expanded access (Abramoff et al., 2022). It is yet to be seen how commercial health insurance and governments outside of the United States will develop their own processes to reimburse for AI-based devices or platforms.

Challenges and Pitfalls

While a few AI solutions are implemented now, most face the challenge of growth and scalability. Some reasons are related to the reproducibility of results and challenges with the generalizability of the solutions in general populations.

In a study of a deep learning system, 7940 patients were screened for diabetic retinopathy, 7651 (96.3%) patients were eligible for study analysis, and 2412 (31.5%) patients were referred for diabetic retinopathy, diabetic macular edema, ungradable images, or low visual acuity (Ruamviboonsuk et al., 2022). For vision-threatening diabetic retinopathy, the deep-learning system had an accuracy of 94.7% compared to the retina specialist over-readers, who had an accuracy of 93.5%. Both the positive predictive value (PPV) and the negative predictive value (NPV) for the deep learning system were greater than over-readers, 79.2% compared with 75.6% and 95.5% compared with 92.4%, respectively.

In this screening program, patient data was managed entirely with paper-based records, with no system to track completed patient referrals. The absence of a digitized system slowed down the deep-learning system-based screening process (e.g., manual image upload was necessary) and hindered measuring its effect on referral adherence rates (i.e., no historical data to compare with). The authors concluded that a deep learning system could deliver real-time diabetic retinopathy detection capability similar to retina specialists in community-based screening settings, but the socio-environmental factors and workflows must be taken into consideration when implementing a deep learning system within a large-scale screening program, especially in low-middle-income countries (LMIC).

The reproducibility challenge in AI has been recognized not only in healthcare but also in non-healthcare settings. Despite a large number of medical machine learning–based algorithms in development, few randomized controlled trials (RCTs) for these technologies have been conducted. Of published RCTs, most did not fully adhere to accepted reporting guidelines and had limited inclusion of participants from underrepresented minority groups (Plana et al., 2022). Notably, only 1.3% of research and 0.6% of mature research involved an author from a low- to low-middle-income country (Zhang et al., 2022).

In a systematic review, the search yielded 19,737 articles, of which 41 RCTs involved a median of 294 participants (range: 17–2,488 participants). A total of 16 RCTs (39%) were published in 2021, 21 (51%) were conducted at single sites, and 15 (37%) involved endoscopy (Plana et al., 2022). None of the trials adhered to CONSORT-AI standards, with reasons such as not assessing poor-quality or unavailable input data (38 trials [93%]), not analyzing performance errors (38 [93%]), and not including a statement regarding code or algorithm availability (37 [90%]). The overall risk of bias was high (17% of the trials), and of the 11 trials (27%) that reported race and ethnicity data, the median proportion of participants from underrepresented minority groups was 21% only (range, 0%–51%).

Another important aspect of the implementation and sustainability of these AI algorithms in healthcare is the ability to prove cost-effectiveness. While most of these algorithms have only been implemented in the last few years, we are seeing cost-effective analysis, including direct cost savings and the impact of their use on patients' quality-adjusted life years (QALY). In an analysis of AI-guided colonoscopy as a screening tool compared with no screening, the authors found a 4.8% incremental gain in the relative reduction of colorectal cancer incidence using AI tools (48.9%) when compared with colonoscopy without guidance (44.2%). They also found a 3.6% incremental gain in relative risk reduction of mortality when screening was done with AI guidance (52.3%) compared with colonoscopy screening with no AI (48.7%). AI detection tools decreased the discounted costs per screened individual from $3400 to $3343 (savings of $57 per individual). When extrapolated to the US population level, the implementation of AI detection during colonoscopy screening resulted in an additional yearly prevention of 7194 colorectal cancer cases and 2089 related deaths and yearly savings of US$290 million. The authors concluded that their findings suggest that implementing AI detection tools in colonoscopy screening is a cost-saving strategy to further reduce colorectal cancer incidence and mortality (Areia et al., 2022).

In a recent study of various applications of AI as a diagnostic-support system, using simulations, both cost savings and the impact on QALY were analyzed. In dermatology, AI showed mean costs of $750 and was associated with 86.5 QALYs, whereas the control showed higher costs of $759 (95% CI, $618–$970) with similar QALY outcomes. In dentistry, AI accumulated costs were $429, with 62.4 years per tooth retention, whereas the control was associated with a higher cost of $458 and fewer tooth retention years (60.9 years). In ophthalmology, AI accrued costs of $559, 95% at 8.4 QALYs, although the control was less expensive at $533 and associated with similar QALYs. Such studies are important in defining the value of AI-based delivery of care and are only likely to grow with the real-world adoption of these systems and devices (Gomez Rossi, Rojas-Perilla, Krois, & Schwendicke, 2022).

Beyond the development of AI algorithms, there is growing evidence of the need to incorporate human factors engineering and adaptive human–computer interfaces for ease of use. Similar to FDA requirements of usability and feasibility studies for approvals, user testing and continuous improvement of the interfaces that deliver decisions to clinicians are equally important to have acceptance and use in the clinical workspace.

Adams et al. examined the association between patient outcomes and provider interaction with a deployed machine learning model-based sepsis alert system called the targeted real-time early warning system (TREWS). Their study focused our analysis on 6,877 patients with sepsis who were identified by the alert before the initiation of antibiotic therapy. Adjusting for patient acuity, patients in the group whose alert was confirmed by a clinician within three hours of the alert had a reduced in-hospital mortality rate (3.3%), organ failure, and length of stay compared with patients whose alert was not confirmed by a clinician within three hours. Improvements in mortality rate (4.5%) and organ failure were larger among those patients who were additionally flagged as high risk. They also found that patients with sepsis who had their alert evaluated and confirmed within

3 hours had a 1.85 hour lower median time from alert to first antibiotic order, which probably played a significant role in improved outcomes (Adams et al., 2022).

In another study for the validation of an AI algorithm, the hypotension prediction index (HPI), which predicts hypotension in patients undergoing surgery, was evaluated; the prediction of the algorithm was accurate, but the adoption of its guidance by clinicians was suboptimal. Among the 214 enrolled patients, guidance was provided for 105 (49%). The median time-weighted average mean arterial pressure less than 65 mmHg was 0.14 in guided patients versus 0.14 mmHg in unguided patients, $P = 0.757$. Index guidance, therefore, did not reduce the amount of hypotension to less than 65 mmHg. In the post hoc, guidance was associated with less hypotension when the analysis was restricted to episodes during which clinicians intervened, suggesting that following the guidance could possibly have had an impact on the prevention of hypotension (Maheshwari et al., 2020).

Evaluation Methods

With a rapidly growing number of AI algorithms, it is important to have evaluation methods that provide guidance for their evaluation. While evaluation methods for AI have been developed by various governmental and research groups in healthcare (CONSORT-AI, SPIRIT-AI), they focus on the reporting of research findings and regulatory aspects. Recently, an international multi-stakeholder group led by Vasey et al. developed a consensus-based reporting guideline called the Developmental and Exploratory Clinical Investigations of Decision Support Systems Driven by Artificial Intelligence (DECIDE-AI) (Vasey et al., 2021). They conducted a two-round, modified Delphi process to collect and analyze expert opinion on the reporting of early clinical evaluation of AI systems. The DECIDE-AI reporting guideline comprises 17 AI-specific reporting items (made of 28 subitems) and 10 generic reporting items. By providing an actionable checklist of minimal reporting items, the DECIDE-AI guideline will facilitate the appraisal of these studies of early-stage clinical studies of AI-based decision support systems in healthcare and the replicability of their findings.

Guidance regarding the assessment of the translational aspects of AI systems, such as safety, utility, clinical adoption, and implementation, has also been recently proposed by another international group (Reddy et al., 2021). They developed a translationally focused evaluation framework termed "Translational Evaluation of Healthcare AI (TEHAI)" based on a critical review of literature focused on health technology evaluation and translational principles to identify key reporting components. These were independently reviewed for consensus inclusion in a final framework by an international panel of experts. The proposed guidelines include three main components – capability, utility, and adoption – with their 15 subcomponents, which can be applied at any stage of the development and deployment of the AI system using a checklist (Figure 8.2).

Three main components – capability, utility and adoption – with 15 subcomponents. The components and associated subcomponents are represented in the same color. Subcomponents with cross-relationships are linked by bold arrows. AI, artificial intelligence; TEHAI, Translational Evaluation of Healthcare AI.

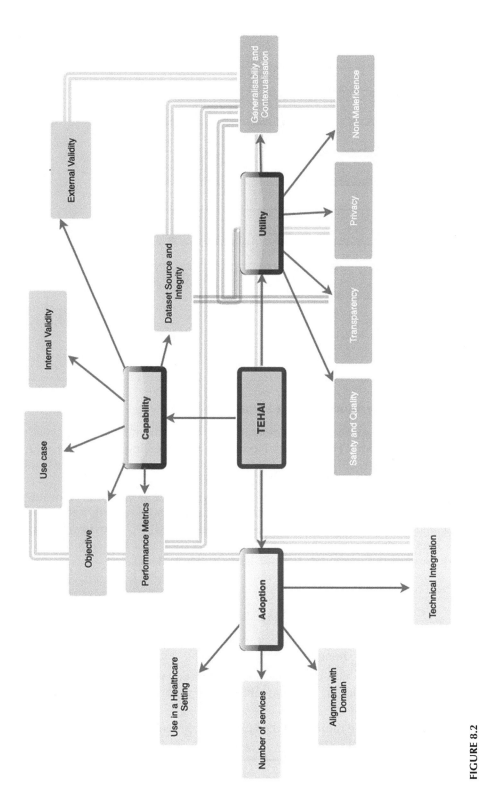

FIGURE 8.2
Translational evaluation of healthcare AI.
(Source: Reddy et al., 2021.)

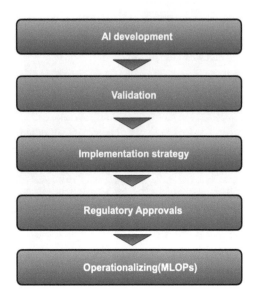

FIGURE 8.3
Roadmap for AI implementation in healthcare.

Roadmap for AI Implementation in Healthcare

Key aspects of the roadmap for AI implementation in healthcare do not differ greatly, except for some modifications, but they need to include the following (Figure 8.3): (1) AI development, (2) validation, (3) implementation strategy, (4) regulatory approvals, and (5) machine learning operations (MLOps) (Miclaus et al., 2020).

While in healthcare, the first four of these key aspects have been more vigorously researched and implemented, MLOps, which is generally a more recently established and evolving field of science, is just starting to be looked into. MLOps provides a framework for the large-scale implementation of AI, which is what will be required for the continuous deployment of AI models (John, Olsson, & Bosch, 2021).

SUMMARY

- Research in AI applications for healthcare has grown exponentially, but mainly in areas using image-based data
- Governmental and non-governmental agencies have created guidelines and frameworks for the evaluation of AI algorithm evaluation in healthcare.
- There is an increasing number of the US FDA-approved algorithms available for use in clinical settings.

- Reimbursement pathways and evaluation of return on investment for AI in healthcare applications are evolving.
- Strategies for successful development and to overcome challenges related to sustainable deployment have to include key techniques such as MLOps for the monitoring and maintenance of AI algorithms in healthcare.

REVIEW QUESTIONS

- Which type of AI models have been mostly researched for AI applications in healthcare and why?
- Describe some of the current regulation and its impact on approval of AI in healthcare algorithms.
- Describe some of the key AI in healthcare evaluation frameworks and their key components.
- Describe possible reimbursement models currently in place for AI algorithms in healthcare and how they can be leveraged.
- What are the key focus areas of a strategic plan for the successful deployment of AI algorithms in healthcare?

References

Abedi, V., Goyal, N., Tsivgoulis, G., Hosseinichimeh, N., Hontecillas, R., Bassaganya-Riera, J., ... Liebeskind, D. S. (2017). Novel screening tool for stroke using artificial neural network. *Stroke, 48*(6), 1678–1681.

Abramoff, M. D., Roehrenbeck, C., Trujillo, S., Goldstein, J., Graves, A. S., Repka, M. X., & Silva III, E. Z. (2022). A reimbursement framework for artificial intelligence in Healthcare. *NPJ Digit Med, 5*(1), 72. doi:10.1038/s41746-022-00621-w

Acosta, J. N., Falcone, G. J., Rajpurkar, P., & Topol, E. J. (2022). Multimodal biomedical AI. *Nat Med, 28*(9), 1773–1784. doi:10.1038/s41591-022-01981-2

Adams, R., Henry, K. E., Sridharan, A., Soleimani, H., Zhan, A., Rawat, N., ... Saria, S. (2022). Prospective, multi-site study of patient outcomes after implementation of the TREWS machine learning-based early warning system for sepsis. *Nat Med, 28*(7), 1455–1460. doi:10.1038/s41591-022-01894-0

Areia, M., Mori, Y., Correale, L., Repici, A., Bretthauer, M., Sharma, P., ... Hassan, C. (2022). Cost-effectiveness of artificial intelligence for screening colonoscopy: A modelling study. *Lancet Digit Health, 4*(6), e436–e444. doi:10.1016/S2589-7500(22)00042-5

Callaway, E. (2020). It will change everything: DeepMind's AI makes gigantic leap in solving protein structures. *Nature, 588* (7837), 203–204. doi:10.1038/d41586-020-03348-4

Chatterjee, A., Somayaji, N. R., & Kabakis, I. M. (2019). Abstract WMP16: Artificial intelligence detection of large cerebrovascular vessel occlusion: Nine-month, 650-patient evaluation of the diagnostic accuracy and performance of the Viz. AI LVO algorithm. *Stroke, 50*(Suppl_1), AWMP16.

Chen, J., Lyell, D., Laranjo, L., & Magrabi, F. (2020). Effect of speech recognition on problem solving and recall in consumer digital health tasks: Controlled laboratory experiment. *J Med Internet Res, 22*(6), e14827. doi:10.2196/14827

Chilamkurthy, S., Ghosh, R., Tanamala, S., Biviji, M., Campeau, N. G., Venugopal, V. K., ... Warier, P. (2018). Deep learning algorithms for detection of critical findings in head CT scans: A retrospective study. *Lancet, 392*(10162), 2388–2396. doi:10.1016/s0140-6736(18)31645-3

Fleming, N. (2018). How artificial intelligence is changing drug discovery. *Nature, 557*(7707), S55–s57. doi:10.1038/d41586-018-05267-x

Ghorbani, A., Ouyang, D., Abid, A., He, B., Chen, J. H., Harrington, R. A., ... Zou, J. Y. (2020). Deep learning interpretation of echocardiograms. *NPJ Digit Med, 3*, 10. doi:10.1038/s41746-019-0216-8

Gomez Rossi, J., Rojas-Perilla, N., Krois, J., & Schwendicke, F. (2022). Cost-effectiveness of artificial intelligence as a decision-support system applied to the detection and grading of melanoma, dental caries, and diabetic retinopathy. *JAMA Netw Open, 5*(3), e220269. doi:10.1001/jamanetworkopen.2022.0269

Gomolin, A., Netchiporouk, E., Gniadecki, R., & Litvinov, I. V. (2020). Artificial intelligence applications in dermatology: Where do we stand? *Front Med (Lausanne), 7*, 100. doi:10.3389/fmed.2020.00100

Graham, S., Depp, C., Lee, E. E., Nebeker, C., Tu, X., Kim, H. C., & Jeste, D. V. (2019). Artificial intelligence for mental health and mental illnesses: An overview. *Curr Psychiatry Rep, 21*(11), 116. doi:10.1007/s11920-019-1094-0

Gupta, R., Kurc, T., Sharma, A., Almeida, J. S., & Saltz, J. (2019). The emergence of pathomics. *Current Pathobiology Reports, 7*(3), 73–84. doi:10.1007/s40139-019-00200-x

Hand, S. (2018). IDx-DR becomes first FDA-approved AI-based diagnostic for diabetic retinopathy. Retrieved from https://xtalks.com/idx-dr-becomes-first-fda-approved-ai-based-diagnostic-for-diabetic-retinopathy-1274/

He, J., Baxter, S. L., Xu, J., Xu, J., Zhou, X., & Zhang, K. (2019). The practical implementation of artificial intelligence technologies in medicine. *Nat Med, 25*(1), 30–36. doi:10.1038/s41591-018-0307-0

Henstock, P. V. (2019). Artificial intelligence for pharma: Time for internal investment. *Trends Pharmacol Sci, 40*(8), 543–546. doi:10.1016/j.tips.2019.05.003

John, M. M., Olsson, H. H., & Bosch, J. (2021). *Towards MLOps: A framework and maturity model. Paper presented at the 2021 47th Euromicro Conference on Software Engineering and Advanced Applications (SEAA).*

Kasasbeh, A. S., Christensen, S., Parsons, M. W., Campbell, B., Albers, G. W., & Lansberg, M. G. (2019). Artificial neural network computer tomography perfusion prediction of ischemic core. *Stroke, 50*(6), 1578–1581. doi:10.1161/strokeaha.118.022649

Liu, J. A., Yang, I. Y., & Tsai, E. B. (2022). Artificial intelligence (AI) for lung nodules, from the AJR special series on AI applications. *AJR Am J Roentgenol, 219*(5), 703–712. doi:10.2214/ajr.22.27487

Madani, A., Arnaout, R., Mofrad, M., & Arnaout, R. (2018). Fast and accurate view classification of echocardiograms using deep learning. *NPJ Digit Med, 1*. doi:10.1038/s41746-017-0013-1

Maheshwari, K., Shimada, T., Yang, D., Khanna, S., Cywinski, J. B., Irefin, S. A., ... Sessler, D. I. (2020). Hypotension prediction index for prevention of hypotension during moderate- to high-risk noncardiac surgery. *Anesthesiology, 133*(6), 1214–1222. doi:10.1097/ALN.0000000000003557

Mastrodicasa, D., Codari, M., Bäumler, K., Sandfort, V., Shen, J., Mistelbauer, G., ... Fleischmann, D. (2022). Artificial intelligence applications in aortic dissection imaging. *Semin Roentgenol, 57*(4), 357–363. doi:10.1053/j.ro.2022.07.001

Miclaus, T., Valla, V., Koukoura, A., Nielsen, A. A., Dahlerup, B., Tsianos, G. I., & Vassiliadis, E. (2020). Impact of design on medical device safety. *Ther Innov Regul Sci*, 54(4), 839–849. doi:10.1007/s43441-019-00022-4

Muehlematter, U. J., Daniore, P., & Vokinger, K. N. (2021). Approval of artificial intelligence and machine learning-based medical devices in the USA and Europe (2015–20): A comparative analysis. *Lancet Digit Health*, 3(3), e195–e203. doi:10.1016/s2589-7500(20)30292-2

Narang, A., Bae, R., Hong, H., Thomas, Y., Surette, S., Cadieu, C., ... Thomas, J. D. (2021). Utility of a deep-learning algorithm to guide novices to acquire echocardiograms for limited diagnostic use. *JAMA Cardiol*, 6(6), 624–632. doi:10.1001/jamacardio.2021.0185

Perez, M. V., Mahaffey, K. W., Hedlin, H., Rumsfeld, J. S., Garcia, A., Ferris, T., ... Apple Heart Study, I. (2019). Large-scale assessment of a smartwatch to identify atrial fibrillation. *N Engl J Med*, 381(20), 1909–1917. doi:10.1056/NEJMoa1901183

Plana, D., Shung, D. L., Grimshaw, A. A., Saraf, A., Sung, J. J. Y., & Kann, B. H. (2022). Randomized clinical trials of machine learning interventions in health care: A systematic review. *JAMA Netw Open*, 5(9), e2233946. doi:10.1001/jamanetworkopen.2022.33946

Polesie, S., Gillstedt, M., Kittler, H., Lallas, A., Tschandl, P., Zalaudek, I., & Paoli, J. (2020). Attitudes towards artificial intelligence within dermatology: An international online survey. *Br J Dermatol*, 183(1), 159–161. doi:10.1111/bjd.18875

Reddy, S., Rogers, W., Makinen, V. P., Coiera, E., Brown, P., Wenzel, M., ... Kelly, B. (2021). Evaluation framework to guide implementation of AI systems into healthcare settings. *BMJ Health Care Inform*, 28(1). doi:10.1136/bmjhci-2021-100444

Ruamviboonsuk, P., Tiwari, R., Sayres, R., Nganthavee, V., Hemarat, K., Kongprayoon, A., ... Webster, D. R. (2022). Real-time diabetic retinopathy screening by deep learning in a multisite national screening programme: A prospective interventional cohort study. *Lancet Digit Health*, 4(4), e235–e244. doi:10.1016/s2589-7500(22)00017-6

Safran, T., Viezel-Mathieu, A., Corban, J., Kanevsky, A., Thibaudeau, S., & Kanevsky, J. (2018). Machine learning and melanoma: The future of screening. *J Am Acad Dermatol*, 78(3), 620–621. doi:10.1016/j.jaad.2017.09.055

Shur, J. D., Doran, S. J., Kumar, S., Ap Dafydd, D., Downey, K., O'Connor, J. P. B., ... Orton, M. R. (2021). Radiomics in oncology: A practical guide. *Radiographics*, 41(6), 1717–1732. doi:10.1148/rg.2021210037

Soun, J. E., Chow, D. S., Nagamine, M., Takhtawala, R. S., Filippi, C. G., Yu, W., & Chang, P. D. (2021). Artificial intelligence and acute stroke imaging. *AJNR Am J Neuroradiol*, 42(1), 2–11. doi:10.3174/ajnr.A6883

Spadaccini, M., Iannone, A., Maselli, R., Badalamenti, M., Desai, M., Chandrasekar, V. T., ... Repici, A. (2021). Computer-aided detection versus advanced imaging for detection of colorectal neoplasia: A systematic review and network meta-analysis. *Lancet Gastroenterol Hepatol*, 6(10), 793–802. doi:10.1016/s2468-1253(21)00215-6

Tang, F. H., Ng, D. K., & Chow, D. H. (2011). An image feature approach for computer-aided detection of ischemic stroke. *Comput Biol Med*, 41(7), 529–536. doi:10.1016/j.compbiomed.2011.05.001

Vasey, B., Clifton, D. A., Collins, G. S., Denniston, A. K., Faes, L., Geerts, B. F., ... The, D.-A. I. S. G. (2021). DECIDE-AI: New reporting guidelines to bridge the development-to-implementation gap in clinical artificial intelligence. *Nature Medicine*, 27(2), 186–187. doi:10.1038/s41591-021-01229-5

Yao, X., McCoy, R. G., Friedman, P. A., Shah, N. D., Barry, B. A., Behnken, E. M., ... Noseworthy, P. A. (2020). ECG AI-guided screening for low ejection fraction (EAGLE): Rationale and design of a pragmatic cluster randomized trial. *Am Heart J*, 219, 31–36. doi:10.1016/j.ahj.2019.10.007

You, Y., & Gui, X. (2020). Self-diagnosis through AI-enabled Chatbot-based symptom checkers: User experiences and design considerations. *AMIA Annu Symp Proc, 2020*, 1354–1363.

Zakhem, G. A., Fakhoury, J. W., Motosko, C. C., & Ho, R. S. (2021). Characterizing the role of dermatologists in developing artificial intelligence for assessment of skin cancer. *J Am Acad Dermatol, 85*(6), 1544–1556. doi:10.1016/j.jaad.2020.01.028

Zhang, J., Whebell, S., Gallifant, J., Budhdeo, S., Mattie, H., Lertvittayakumjorn, P., ... Teo, J. T. (2022). An interactive dashboard to track themes, development maturity, and global equity in clinical artificial intelligence research. *Lancet Digit Health, 4*(4), e212–e213. doi:10.1016/S2589-7500(22)00032-2

Index

Pages in *italics* refer to figures and pages in **bold** refer to tables.

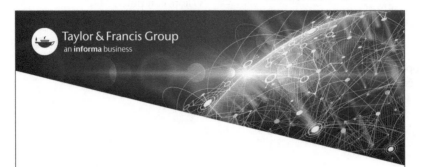